The Complete Idiot's Reference Card

cut here

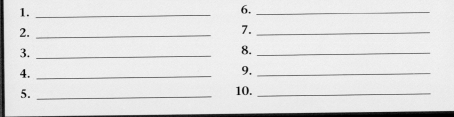

The Top 10 Bad Habits Anyone Can Have, According to the Expert—You!

Everyone has a list of the habits they think are the worst ones known to humankind. Those cravings, tendencies, and compulsions that just drive them nuts. Which habits, as a rule, drive *you* crazy?

1. _____
2. _____
3. _____
4. _____
5. _____

6. _____
7. _____
8. _____
9. _____
10. _____

How My Own Bad Habits Make Me Feel

Identifying habits you'd classify as "bad" is just the starting point, because, after all, you're ready to break your *own* bad habits. You know it's time to change if you've checked off more boxes in column A than in column B.

COLUMN A
- ❏ Stressed out
- ❏ Annoyed
- ❏ Overwhelmed
- ❏ Bored
- ❏ Unworthy

COLUMN B
- ❏ Relaxed
- ❏ Satisfied
- ❏ In control
- ❏ Engaged
- ❏ Self-confident

Using the Daily Habit Log

Use the Daily Habit Log on the reverse side of this card to help you get a fix on the how, why, when, and where of your personal bad habits. At the end of the week, take a good look at the information you've recorded and see what clues it reveals about your bad habit and why you do it. Good luck!

alpha
books

My Daily Habit Log

MONDAY

Time: _____
Habit: _____
Activity: _____
Feeling: _____

Time: _____
Habit: _____
Activity: _____
Feeling: _____

Time: _____
Habit: _____
Activity: _____
Feeling: _____

Time: _____
Habit: _____
Activity: _____
Feeling: _____

TUESDAY

Time: _____
Habit: _____
Activity: _____
Feeling: _____

Time: _____
Habit: _____
Activity: _____
Feeling: _____

Time: _____
Habit: _____
Activity: _____
Feeling: _____

Time: _____
Habit: _____
Activity: _____
Feeling: _____

WEDNESDAY

Time: _____
Habit: _____
Activity: _____
Feeling: _____

Time: _____
Habit: _____
Activity: _____
Feeling: _____

Time: _____
Habit: _____
Activity: _____
Feeling: _____

Time: _____
Habit: _____
Activity: _____
Feeling: _____

THURSDAY

Time: _____
Habit: _____
Activity: _____
Feeling: _____

Time: _____
Habit: _____
Activity: _____
Feeling: _____

Time: _____
Habit: _____
Activity: _____
Feeling: _____

Time: _____
Habit: _____
Activity: _____
Feeling: _____

FRIDAY

Time: _____
Habit: _____
Activity: _____
Feeling: _____

Time: _____
Habit: _____
Activity: _____
Feeling: _____

Time: _____
Habit: _____
Activity: _____
Feeling: _____

Time: _____
Habit: _____
Activity: _____
Feeling: _____

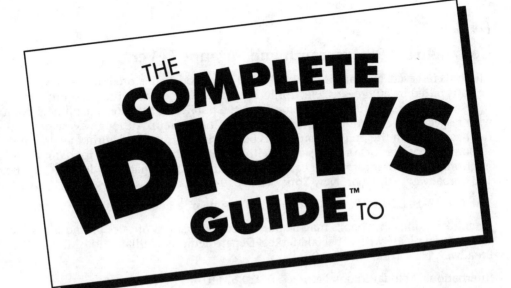

THE
COMPLETE
IDIOT'S
GUIDE™ TO

Breaking Bad
Habits

*by Suzanne LeVert
and Gary McClain, Ph.D.*

alpha
books

A Division of Macmillan Reference USA
A Simon & Schuster Macmillan Company
1633 Broadway, New York, NY 10019

For Bob

Copyright©1998 Amaranth and Suzanne LeVert

THE COMPLETE IDIOT'S GUIDE name and design are trademarks of Macmillan, Inc.

Macmillan Publishing books may be purchased for business or sales promotional use. For information please write: Special Markets Department, Macmillan Publishing USA, 1633 Broadway, New York, NY 10019.

International Standard Book Number: 0-02-862110-7
Library of Congress Catalog Card Number: 97-80969

99 98   8 7 6 5 4 3 2 1

Interpretation of the printing code: the rightmost number of the first series of numbers is the year of the book's printing; the rightmost number of the second series of numbers is the number of the book's printing. For example, a printing code of 98-1 shows that the first printing occurred in 1998.

Printed in the United States of America

Alpha Development Team

Brand Manager
Kathy Nebenhaus

Executive Editor
Gary M. Krebs

Managing Editor
Bob Shuman

Senior Editor
Nancy Mikhail

Development Editor
Jennifer Perillo

Editorial Assistant
Maureen Horn

Production Team

Development Editor/Book Producer
Lee Ann Chearney/Amaranth

Production Editor
Chris Van Camp

Copy Editor
Michael Cunningham

Cover Designer
Mike Freeland

Cartoonist
Judd Winick

Designer
Glenn Larsen

Indexer
Chris Barrick

Proofreading/Layout
Angela Perry, Daniela Raderstorf

Contents at a Glance

Contents

Foreword

Jiggling your knee under the desk. Drinking a little too much at the office party. Biting your nails. Watching television from morning 'til night. There are more bad habits than any of us can count, and new ones arise every day. Ten years ago, who would have thought there would be support groups for people addicted to chatting on the Internet?

No matter what form they take, bad habits are, by their very nature, disruptive—to your daily life, to your relationships, to your self-esteem. The effect they have may be subtle or dramatic, depending on the habit and your lifestyle. But if you're reading this book, my guess is that you've decided that you or someone you love has a bad habit disruptive enough to warrant breaking it.

Unfortunately, that's easier said than done. In my experience, bad habits have deep roots. They involve the total personality, the unconscious as well as the conscious. Bad habits are the unhealthy ways we choose to release anxiety or stress, ways that we usually learn in very early childhood and carry with us through much of our adult lives—until we finally take the bull by the horns and regain control of our lives.

This book shows you how to do just that—how to break the negative patterns of behavior that have been holding you back. Step by step, Suzanne LeVert and Gary McClain, Ph.D., show you how to identify your bad habit, understand the role it plays in your life, and then learn how to break it.

Whether you want to:

➤ Quit smoking

➤ Stop overspending

➤ Communicate more directly

➤ Turn off the computer or the television

➤ Develop healthier eating habits

➤ Take control over any negative behavior pattern

this book is for you. Indeed, if you're ready—or even close to ready—to break your bad habit, I suggest you do two things: First, read this book and take its positive message to heart. You *can* change your behavior and leave your bad habit behind. Second, practice the techniques outlined here. You'll learn both general principles behind the process of change and specific methods for breaking bad habits.

If you're really interested in changing for good, this book will show you the way. Read on!

Jane Ferber, M.D.

Dr. Ferber is an assistant clinical professor of psychiatry at Columbia University College of Physicians and Surgeons, and associate director of psychiatric residency training at Creedmoor Psychiatric Center. She is an individual and family therapist who practices in New Rochelle, New York, and the author of A Woman Doctor's Guide to Depression *(Hyperion, 1997).*

Introduction

You've got one, don't you? Or know someone who does?

Bad habits are like death and taxes: Everybody has experience with them and that experience tends to be negative! But don't be embarrassed or frustrated. We've written this book to let you know there's light at the end of the unpleasant bad habit tunnel, and we're here to show you the way out.

We learned a lot by writing this book, and we each came to the project with an interesting contribution to make. Gary McClain, Ph.D., has years of experience as a psychologist helping people develop more positive, healthier coping skills. Suzanne LeVert's interviewed hundreds of men and women and researched virtually every bad habit during her career as a health writer. We both felt excited about communicating helpful, accurate information that could help people achieve success in breaking their bad habits.

What surprised both of us, however, was how often we came face to face with our own bad habits as we wrote this book together. "Oh dear, I do that, too," was an oft-heard phrase in our many conversations. We were also surprised at how many bad habits we shared—procrastination mixed with perfection and a tendency to overeat when under stress, to name just two. In a way, writing about these topics helped us recognize, and then begin to change, the negative behaviors affecting our *own* lives.

Another thing we learned by writing this book is how different the process of change is for everyone who embarks upon it. You might find it best to quit smoking cold turkey and do just great, for example, while your neighbor weans himself with six or eight weeks on the nicotine patch. You might discover that you overeat because of a long-standing self-esteem issue that first arose in childhood, while your best friend didn't start to have a problem with food until becoming overwhelmed by the stress of a new job.

In other words, we learned that there are no hard and fast rules that would work for every person who reads this book. That's why we decided to provide insight and advice that could apply to as wide a range of people—and habits—as possible.

The fun part was discovering how much and how often we could draw from our family and friends for examples and perspective. "Yes, Mom or Sis or Best Buddy, that's you in the book," we can say with a chuckle—and hopefully receive a chuckle in return! (Of course, when appropriate, names have been changed to protect the innocent...) Because that's the thing about bad habits: It's actually pretty hard to find someone *without* one or two they could benefit from breaking.

In the end, the most exciting thing about writing this book was knowing we'd be providing people just like you with information that could really change their lives for the better.

How to Use This Book

We're gonna be up front with you, right from the start. This book provides you with all the information you'll need to get started on breaking your bad habit, but it isn't going to be easy. And, quite honestly, you just might not find *all* the help you need here. We don't delve into the world of hard-core addictions, nor do we expect that our relatively short chapter on food, as an example, will answer all of your questions about the good and bad habits related to nutrition, diet, and fitness.

But we can make this promise: If you read this book and follow our suggestions, you'll gain a tremendous amount of insight into your negative behavior, discover the techniques you'll need to change it, and—if the problem is bigger than you imagined—learn what your next step should be. And we *guarantee* you'll have some fun getting there!

Consider this book as:

> ➤ An entry into the subject of bad habits and the process of breaking them.

> ➤ A motivational aid to encourage you along the way.

> ➤ A starting point for issues and ideas you want to explore further.

We've divided this book into six sections, each of which explores a different aspect of bad habits and how to break them. At the heart of every chapter, however, is one basic message: You've got the power to gain control over your bad habit, no matter what it is. When you do that, you boost your self-esteem while clearing away an obstacle that'd otherwise prevent you from meeting present and future goals. Here's what you find:

Part 1, "Over and Over Again," explores the basics of bad habits: what role they play in your life, how they develop, the damage they do to your goals and sense of self-esteem, and the many forms they can take. Self-tests and exercises help you identify the habits—good and bad—in your life, while the text gently guides you toward a greater understanding of your lifestyle and its effects on your behavior.

Part 2, "Just Say No!" serves as a step-by-step outline of the process of change. It starts by helping you pinpoint your negative behavior and when and why it occurs, then moves you into a discussion of the risks (how it damages your self-esteem or undermines your goals) and the benefits (the immediate gratification and release of stress) your bad habit offers. Once you've decided that the risks outweigh the benefits, we help you prepare yourself and your environment for the changes you're about to make. We give you clear-cut strategies and techniques to break your bad habit once and for all.

Part 3, "Resist Those Cravings," explores the world of substances—alcohol, nicotine, caffeine, and food—and the powerful hold they can have over the average person. With frequent warnings about the signs of addiction, we offer tips to help you break free from the common problems connected to substances: Drink a little too much at social activities? We show how to avoid that trap next time. Still smoking? We provide the most up-to-date techniques available to help you quit. If caffeine gives you the jitters, you'll learn how to cut down or eliminate it from your diet. And when it comes to your relationship to food, we explore the most common dietary pitfalls and how you can learn to avoid them.

Part 4, "Stop Driving Me (and Everyone Else) Crazy!" shows how certain bad habits profoundly affect the relationships in your life. We discuss how lying, losing your temper, and procrastinating can get in the way of positive, dynamic associations with lovers, friends, and family members. We also provide tips that will help you break those undermining patterns and establish healthy communication with the other people in your life.

Part 5, "Calm Those Compulsions," helps you identify the automatic and habitual behaviors you just can't resist. These habits range from the physical ones, like knuckle-cracking and nail-biting, to the active, like being too neat and meticulous (or being too sloppy!), overspending, and gambling. We also discuss a relatively new compulsion: logging on to the Internet and losing yourself there for hours longer than you can afford. Television and telephone compulsions are also covered.

Part 6, "Bad Habits and the Big Picture," takes the information you've learned throughout the book one step further. If someone you love has a bad habit, we show you the best ways to help them, while avoiding approaches that might raise their defenses. In some cases, you may need further help and support from physicians, mental health professionals, and support groups, and we let you know when and how to reach out for that help. Finally, we help you celebrate the remarkable progress you've made in understanding how your bad habit affects your life and in making positive, lasting changes.

Extras

In addition to all that carefully constructed information, you'll find sidebars designed to make identifying and breaking your bad habit even easier. These boxes feature easily digestible tidbits of information you're sure to find interesting. Here's what to look for:

Cold Turkey

Warnings! The information provided in these boxes helps you steer clear of negative behaviors, substances, or ways of thinking that will get in the way of your process of change.

One Day at a Time

Tips! In these boxes, we offer you advice on healthy ways to break your bad habit, generally reinforcing the information you find in the text.

A New Angle

Tidbits! Here, you'll read about interesting studies, statistics, and viewpoints that relate to bad habits and the best ways to break them.

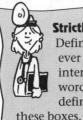

Strictly Speaking

Definitions! Whenever we introduce an interesting or obscure word or term, we define it in one of these boxes.

Special Thanks from the Publisher to the Technical Reviewer

Our thanks to Marci Pliskin, CSW, ACSW, a psychotherapist in Seattle, Washington. Ms. Pliskin's expertise has provided valuable insights and direction to the book. Her patience, talent, and enthusiasm for this project are greatly appreciated!

Acknowledgments

We have lots of people to thank for helping us with this book, including, first and foremost, our friends and families. Not only did they provide us with moral support and encouragement, they also supplied a number of anecdotes and case studies that added a great deal to the book!

We owe an enormous debt of gratitude to Lee Ann Chearney, creative director of Amaranth, our editor and life-support system. She saw us through the process with grace and good humor, while adding significant insight into each and every chapter. Without her, the book would probably lack some vital focus, and would certainly be twice as long!

Lisa Lenard and Eve Adamson, two excellent writers and researchers, were instrumental in the writing and editing of several chapters in the book. Their talent and professionalism, as well as their contributions, are greatly appreciated. We also want to thank Roz Kramer, artist-extraordinare, who helped many visual elements—including the handy Daily Habit Logs!—come alive for readers.

Finally, our gratitude goes out all the good people at Macmillan who made this book possible, including Kathy Nebenhaus, Gary Krebs, Robert Shuman, Maureen Horn, and Chris Van Camp. Their patience and faith kept us going!

Part 1
Over and Over Again

"Habit? I don't have no stinkin' bad habit! If my friends can't stand my knuckle-cracking, they can just leave the room. It's their problem, not mine."

"You mean being chronically late with my sales reports is a bad habit? And it's kept me from getting a promotion?"

"I can stop any time I want. As many times as I want. But can I really stop forever?"

Sound familiar? Could you have a bad habit that interferes with your goals and sense of self-esteem?

Before you can even think about breaking your bad habit(s), it's important to gain a deeper understanding of the role that habits play in your life. Some habits may be positive and healthful—like brushing your teeth three times a day, or getting to the gym on a regular basis—while others may be disruptive or downright dangerous. Finding out what bad habits you have, and how they affect your life, is the first step in the process of change.

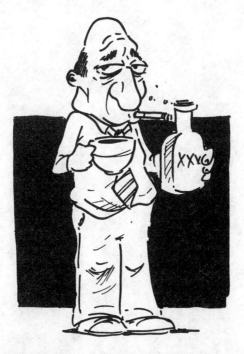

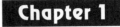

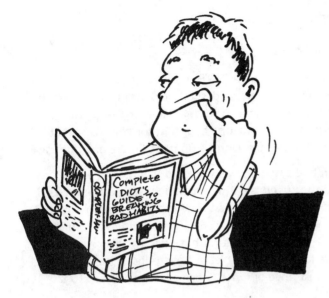

Chapter 1

What Is a Bad Habit?

In This Chapter

➤ Understanding habits, good and bad

➤ Identifying your lifestyle pitfalls

➤ Discovering how habits interfere with your life

➤ Finding the courage to change

Does it seem like this book was written just for you? Do you feel like a complete idiot because you can't stop smoking no matter how hard (or how often) you try? Or do you feel helpless against the need to spin the dice or play the slots every Friday night? Do you kick yourself when you look down at your hands and see fingernails that look as if tiny animals have been gnawing at them? Or maybe you've missed the start of the last seven movies because you just can't manage to: a) find your wallet, b) finish up at work on time, or c) remember which girlfriend you made the date with and what you told the other one?

If so, you're not alone. Bad habits are as common as mosquito bites in the summer—and just as annoying. Most of us have at least one tendency or behavior we'd like to change, and at least one that drives someone in our lives to distraction. Maybe you've only just now realized that something you do on a regular basis interferes with your goals, your self-image, or your health. Or maybe you've known you've had this habit for quite a while, but never knew how to change. If you're like most people you not only know about your bad habit, you've also tried and failed—and tried and failed again and again—to quit it.

Before we go any further, believe this much: You are NOT an idiot. Nor are you too weak, too stubborn, too old, too young, too busy, too stressed, too bored, or just plain too in love with your bad habit to stop. In fact, you've taken a remarkable first step just by picking up this book. And if a "well-meaning" someone bought it for you, you've still managed to take that first step by reading this far. Don't stop now. You're on your way.

We're not going to lie to you. It won't be easy to break your bad habit, or to add a healthy new one. By its very definition, a *habit* is an ingrained behavior learned over time and with practice. You didn't bite your nails for the first time just yesterday. If you did, it'd be a snap to stop biting them today. Last month wasn't the first time you put off starting the monthly sales report. If it were, you wouldn't have had the very same problem this month, or the month before last. You didn't learn how to lie so seamlessly to your boss or your spouse by doing it just once or twice. Once or twice became 10, 20, 100 times—and therein lies the problem.

We decided to write this book because we want to help you kick your bad habits. (Yes, it *is* possible!) Everyone has them, and everyone wants to get rid of them; it's a universal human condition. You might even find yourself establishing some *good* habits, or at least learning more about why you do things the way you do. As a writer, Suzanne has got some bad habits of her own, some stylistic (e.g., writing sentences long enough to rival

Strictly Speaking

A **habit** is a routine practice, something you do the same way, usually for the same reason until it becomes second nature. A habit is neither good nor bad: Its consequences are what define it. A **bad habit** is a tendency or action that hinders or harms you, while a **good habit** is a practice that increases your self-esteem, improves your health, and/or maintains healthy interpersonal relationships.

William Faulkner on a bad day) and others more behavior oriented (e.g., waiting until the last minute before getting started on a project). And writing books about other types of psychological problems, including depression and Attention Deficit Disorder, has given her some insight into the way the human brain establishes behavior problems like bad habits. The other half of this team, psychologist Gary McClain, is shy about revealing his own bad habits, but he *has* shared his many years of experience as a therapist working with people who are struggling to break their own.

In this chapter, the two of us will show you just what a bad habit is, how to differentiate it from a harmless one, and how to start thinking about changing the behavior.

An occasional white lie to help you through an awkward situation may be perfectly acceptable. If your best friend asks you about her new haircut, you don't want to run screaming out into the night even if it does look like something the cat coughed up. Instead, a smile and a "Oh, Tiffany, it's darling!" is the appropriate response. Smoking an occasional cigarette, say one a month, probably wouldn't pose a health risk to you or to the people around you.

But that's not what bad habits are. They aren't occasional and they aren't harmless.

When a Habit Turns Bad

Nine mornings out of ten, Suzanne gets out of bed, turns on the coffee, uses the bathroom, scans the *New York Times* online, finishes her first cup of coffee, jumps in the shower, gets dressed, and goes back to her computer ready to work. In that order, almost every morning, day after day. Her morning routine is a habit, a satisfactory habit that allows her to get important stuff done without having to make decisions before she's completely awake. She doesn't really decide to do it, she just does it.

Most habits are just like Suzanne's morning routine. Not good, not bad. Just habitual. Habits help us establish order and add rhythm to our daily lives. The fact is, we couldn't live without maintaining habits, or at least we couldn't live well. Chaos would reign, especially today, when information comes at us fast and furious, demanding our immediate attention, insisting that we consider its implications and, often, make quick decisions. If we didn't have habits, we'd be thrown headlong into one unfamiliar situation, activity, or thought process after another. As Gary points out, without habits, we wouldn't receive the comfort that comes from the usual, the customary, and the routine.

Think about it. There's nothing special about having that bran muffin with low-fat cream cheese (not butter—never butter!) every weekday morning. You could, of course, get a bagel instead. You like bagels. You eat them on Sundays while you're doing the crossword puzzle. But something about the familiarity of buying the muffin at the stand right near the train station and eating it while you go through your mail at the office comforts you. It feels right.

Is having the same thing for breakfast every morning a *bad* habit? Not unless six bran muffins and a rasher of bacon is what constitutes your daily breakfast. Or unless you are completely unable to function unless you have the *exact* same thing—no substitutions allowed—in which case a run-of-the-mill habit has become an obsession.

Cold Turkey
Do you have persistent, seemingly irresistible, and irrational thoughts or behaviors: "I *must* have a bran muffin for breakfast or I won't be able to speak during today's meeting." "If I don't have this martini, I'll explode." "If I don't buy out Timberland's entire line of hiking boots, it's not worth hiking at all this season." Which of *your* habits are reaching obsession status?

Is eating the same thing for breakfast every morning a *good* habit? Not necessarily, even if it's something good for you. First, there are certainly other foods that would provide you with as much or more nutrition than your beloved bran muffin. Second, most nutritionists recommend varying your diet from day to day to increase the chances that you'll receive all the vitamins and minerals your body needs.

What you've got here, then, is a plain old habit, one that gives you pleasure, doesn't do you harm, and adds some structure to your day. If you think about it, you probably find that you perform several of these little harmless rituals every day.

You'll also—with any luck!—find that you harbor a number of clearly good habits. You might call your mother every Sunday morning, or go to the gym the requisite three times a week, or pay your bills on time every month. Thanks to these and other good habits, you're probably able to look at your life and see a relatively stable, organized, dignified existence.

A New Angle

We call some habits "manners" and, presumably, we learned these conventions at our proverbial mother's knee. Unfortunately, such habits are apparently terribly passé in many sectors of today's society. The habit of sending thank-you notes, saying "excuse me" after belching, and telling your date you're still married were once upon a time routine practices. In our opinion, we could use them all back.

But then there are the *baaad* habits. Some are pretty obvious: cigarette smoking, drinking a little too much (coffee or alcohol), eating too much, being a couch potato, and losing your temper at the drop of a hat to name just a few. Some are only bad habits if you do them in front of people (*any* people, including your spouse), like picking your nose, cracking your knuckles, passing gas, belching. Still others tend to creep up on you: Sure you like to shop, who doesn't? But when you can't pay even the monthly minimum on your credit card and you're considering turning the baby's room into a closet to store your new purchases, you know you're in trouble.

The scary truth about a bad habit is that it can, and often does, start with the very best of intentions, just like the road to hell.

Pick a Habit, Any Habit

"Everything in moderation" became a cliché for a good reason: It's really true, in almost all cases. A clear exception is murder (just one really *is* too many!) and there are no doubt several other crimes and misdemeanors that are completely off-limits.

In most cases, though, balance and moderation are the keys. Suzanne has a couple of friends who love to gamble. They go to Atlantic City on the same middle Saturday every month, to play blackjack at the same table with the same dealer. They take the same amount of money with them ($300, which they lose with astonishing regularity) every time. This night out has become a habit. It isn't a bad habit, because they set limits and stick to them. They enjoy the thrill, then they go home.

Another friend—let's call her Jane—started going to aerobics classes to lose a little weight, gain a little muscle tone, and fill a little free time. Much to her surprise, she liked aerobics. Then she loved aerobics. Three times a week became five times, then six, then sometimes twice a day, an hour each time, kicking, jumping, feeling the burn. When step classes came along, Jane disappeared into the gym and never came out!

But isn't exercise a good thing? Shouldn't we congratulate Jane, and not fault her? Gary points out that, although exercise in moderation is a very good habit, Jane had crossed the line. She now doesn't have much of a life apart from work (which never really interested her much) or the gym. She doesn't have time to go to the movies with friends, or take a continuing education class, or even think about changing careers. She looks great, there's no doubt about it, but the benefits seem to end there.

Jane knows she's got a problem. She's tried to stop or at least limit her time at the gym, but after ten years, exercising so often has become an ingrained habit and, perhaps even a physical addiction. (We'll talk about the fine line between habit and addiction later in this chapter.)

So there you have it. Gambling, known far and wide as a notorious bad habit, may be perfectly benign, even beneficial since it can relieve stress and offer a healthy escape from the real world. But exercise—the one routine most everybody wishes they maintained—can end up being every bit as tedious or even destructive as any other bad habit.

Indeed, virtually any habit can go bad, sort of the way mayonnaise goes bad in the sun. It starts out creamy and delicious, then slowly but surely begins to sour. Once a bad habit takes hold, it can turn destructive.

Top 10 Bad Habits

Have you ever wondered why top ten lists have become as ubiquitous as the Gap? It's probably because they help to systemize our thoughts and sort our priorities. Well, before we make you start thinking about your *own* bad habits, we're going to provide you with a list of what we consider the worst of the bad habits in general. This should get you thinking of what bugs you the most about *other* people—a far safer and more fun way to begin.

1. **Lying.** To us, lying—and not the occasional lie to save your own skin or protect another's feelings—is the most reprehensible habit a person can have. It's lazy, immoral, and destructive.

2. **Being late.** Being late is often passive-aggressive behavior in its purest form. People who are *always* late usually are actually expressing anger.

3. **"Forgetting" and other acts of carelessness.** Ditto.

4. **Knuckle-cracking.** It actually makes us nauseous.

5. **Belching and passing gas.** Rarely, is it absolutely necessary to release gastrointestinal air in public. Very, very, very rarely. (What you do behind closed doors, however, is your own business!)

6. **Obsessive orderliness.** Okay, most of us could stand to clean up our acts a little. However, insisting that the edges of a notebook lay perfectly perpendicular to the edges of the desk is *insane*.

7. **Inability to commit.** To a relationship or anything else. Need we say more?

8. **Being a skinflint.** Fiscal responsibility is admirable. Never opening (or having) your wallet when the check comes is terribly annoying and inconsiderate.

9. **Procrastinating.** We're going to skip this one for now, and get back to it later (Can you tell which habit we relate to most?!)

10. **Cigarette smoking.** No one, not even a die-hard smoker (and can they ever die hard) believes that cigarettes are beneficial or harmless. And we especially hate the way smoke—from someone else's cigarettes—permeates our hair and clothes.

Now, try this exercise. Write down the habits you consider the worst; by doing so, you might gain some perspective on the whole subject. Be honest, even if you have to name a few bad habits, you harbor yourself. In fact, you might want to star the ones that apply to you for future reference!

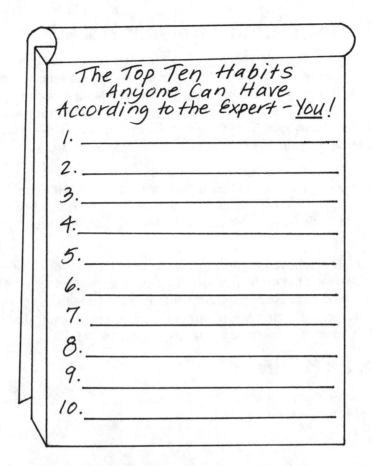

The Top Ten Habits
Anyone Can Have
According to the Expert – You!

1. _____
2. _____
3. _____
4. _____
5. _____
6. _____
7. _____
8. _____
9. _____
10. _____

But You Love Your Daily Rituals

Perhaps by now you see your bad habits with a little more clarity. You can see how they might be doing some damage to at least one aspect of your life.

At the same time, though, you love your habits, don't you? You love even the bad ones. Maybe especially the bad ones because they give you a secret pleasure, a special little thrill. They're your unquestioning, unconditional "friends": The second pint of Häagen-Dazs never pipes up to say, "Haven't you had enough tonight?"

On the other hand, here you are, reading a book about breaking bad habits. Something isn't working anymore, and you're ready (or almost ready!) to make a change. Maybe.

Is Your Life Interfering with Your Habit?

If only you didn't have to pay that pesky gas bill, you'd have enough money to keep the credit card people from calling on an hourly basis. If only your office's "No Smoking" policy weren't so strict, you wouldn't have missed the all-important staff meeting because you were huddled in the vestibule, puffing away. If only your doctor had given you that prescription for valium instead of telling you not to drink a caffeinated soft drink before you went to bed, you wouldn't have to go across the border to Mexico to get those pills to help you sleep.

"If only" is an important concept here in bad habit land. *If only* the world weren't so rigid, we wouldn't have these bad habits. *If only* we didn't have so much stress, so much responsibility, so little time, we'd certainly be able to break a bad habit or two with ease and grace. *If only...*

At some point, however, you're going to have replace "if only" with "but really," as in "I do love my cigarettes, but really they're making me sick," and "I love cracking my knuckles, but really I'd rather have my boy/girlfriend sit in the same room with me on occasion." Unfortunately, the "but really" part of the process sometimes take longer than you may like. Until then, you might just cling to the thought that...

It's Not Me, It's My Life

Your bad habit isn't really a bad habit. Not at all. It's a perfectly natural way of adapting to an incredibly (choose one)...

➤ stressful

➤ busy

➤ boring

world in which you don't (choose one):

➤ look good

➤ feel smart

➤ deserve rewards

If you feel this way, you're not alone. We all suffer the same burdens of modern living: too much to do, too little time, too much stimulation but too little satisfaction, and—most of all—not enough good old-fashioned self-esteem.

Self-Test Challenge: What's Your Lifestyle?

Recognizing the patterns in your daily life, and the amount of stress and pressure you face, will help you better focus on why you've developed your bad habit(s). It may also help you to identify obstacles to change. This quiz will help you do just that.

Part A

1. Does the mere thought of your in-box (proverbial or actual) make your skin itch and your head pound?

2. Does lighting a small fire in Aisle 2 seem like a viable alternative to waiting your turn in line at the grocery checkout?

3. Do you count more sheep than live in New Zealand before closing your eyes at night?

Part B

1. How often do you have time to do absolutely nothing for the whole afternoon?

   (a) once a week

   (b) once a month

   (c) as often as snow falls in Tahiti

2. When did you last spend time in the daylight (besides riding to and from work)?

   (a) just this morning

   (b) a week ago Thursday

   (c) the day Nixon resigned (August 8, 1974)

3. Can you compare the number of entries in your appointment book to:

   (a) the letters of the alphabet

   (b) the listings in *TV Guide*

   (c) the distance in light years from here to Pluto

Part C

1. Do you consider your remote control your best friend?

2. Did the last over-the-top art exhibition/sci-fi flick/literary masterpiece leave you yawning?

3. Is the thrill—of anything—just plain gone?

Part D

1. When asked to describe yourself, do you search for comparisons in:

    (a) *Playboy/Playgirl*

    (b) *Ms./Esquire*

    (c) *Barnyard Animal Review*

2. Is your biggest regret in life that:

    (a) you haven't yet finished your Ph.D.

    (b) they haven't made evening wear yet that flatters you

    (c) you're not someone else

3. If asked to measure your potential for success, what gauge would you use?

    (a) the space shuttle

    (b) a mercury thermometer

    (c) the head of a pin

Answer Key

Part A   If you answered "yes" to one or more of these questions, you probably suffer from stress—the most common malady of the twentieth century and one of the greatest contributors to bad habits. The more stress you have, the more likely you are to rely on some bad habits to relieve it, and the less likely you'll feel able to break them.

Part B   If you circled "C" at least once, you probably don't have enough of what has become a precious commodity—time. And you're not alone. So many of us are pressed for time these days, working hard to make ends meet, and even harder to raise healthy children. Unfortunately, lack of time often leads to bad habits of all kinds.

Part C If you've answered yes to these questions, you're probably just plain bored on top of everything else. Boredom saps energy, inspiration, and commitment, and it can lead to filling in the gaps with harmful, negative behavior. Boredom is one of humankind's greatest—but fortunately most avoidable—enemies.

Part D If you answered "C" to one or more of these questions, your ego could use a little boosting. Low self-esteem is both a cause and a symptom of having a bad habit. You feel depressed or unattractive, so you seek a little solace in a martini (or two) after work. Waking up a little hung-over the next day only makes you feel more depressed and unattractive. One (or two) martinis after work then become three (or four), and pretty soon you've got a full-fledged bad habit—and maybe even a more serious addiction that requires intervention—on your hands.

One Day at a Time
It's important to recognize that it's quite possible to be under stress, extremely busy, and yet terribly bored all at the same time. This combination can be absolutely deadly when it comes to finding the motivation and strength to break a bad habit. In chapters to come, we'll show you how to de-stress while finding meaning and inspiration in your daily life.

Or, Is Your Habit Interfering with Your Life?

Your boss catches you "borrowing" office supplies, more than once. Your investment banking job is on the line because you've pierced one too many body parts and your conservative clients are beginning to look frightened. You're approaching 40 at the speed of light, but still can't say the words "I love you" to the significant other in your life.

Have you discovered that your habit is responsible, at least in some way, for your failure to meet a goal, to live up to your own ideals, or to adhere to the socially accepted rules of professional and personal relationships? Most people don't break a bad habit until they see, clearly and in an up-front and personal way, the harm that it's doing to their lives, the ways it's holding them back. And that's when the process of change really begins.

Since you're reading this book, chances are you're already beginning the process. You can see your bad habit clearly and you're ready to do something about it.

Separating the Good from the Bad

The good news is that you know you have the strength and commitment to *break* your bad habit. How do you know this? Because you've had the strength and commitment to *maintain* it for this long. Okay, it might be easier right now to give into a bad habit than replace it with a new one, but you WILL learn how to give it up.

We know someone who recently quit smoking. James said he didn't do it for health reasons; he did it because he couldn't stand how much of a chore smoking had become. His roommate insisted he go outside to light up, long flights on airplanes became tortuous, and his favorite restaurant relegated him to a tiny table in the back where he sat, either alone or in a cloud of smoke so dense he couldn't see, much less taste, his food.

To keep smoking at work, he walked down three flights of stairs, smoked in the heat, the cold, the snow, the rain, and then walked back up three flights of stairs to his office—sometimes four or five times a day. He learned to scout airports for nooks and crannies "safe" for smoking. He started going to a different restaurant, one with terrible food but a more liberal smoking policy. He did this for years.

Finally, he realized that if he could manage to change his life in such fundamental ways to *maintain* a habit, he really did have the strength and commitment to *break* the habit. And that's just what he did. And you can do it, too.

Walking the Fine Line

Caffeine. Alcohol. Nicotine. These substances are drugs, powerful drugs that cause a physical and psychological dependency we commonly know as *addiction*. Gambling, shopping, compulsive eating, even compulsive cleaning can become not simply bad habits, they can become addictions as well.

Although scientists still don't know exactly what causes an individual to become addicted to a substance or behavior, more and more research points to the involvement of a group of brain chemicals called neurotransmitters. Two of the most "famous" neurotransmitters, and the ones most implicated in most cases of addiction, are endorphins and serotonin.

Many addictions may be fueled, at least in part, to restore a lack of *endorphins* (which are natural pain and stress relievers) or *serotonin* (a brain chemical that influences a wide range of brain activities, including mood, appetite, and pain tolerance). Psychological factors, such as low self-esteem, feelings of powerless, overwhelming states of anxiety and depression also contribute to the development of addictions.

When does a habit become an addiction? That's a good question, and one that everyone—with the help of an experienced physician or therapist—must ask and answer for him or herself.

The subject of addiction is a complex one that goes far beyond the scope of this book. If you think that your habit is truly beyond your power to control, or if it seriously undermines your mental or physical health, seek the advice of a physician right away. (See Appendix A, "More Bad Habit Busters" for some resources that might help.)

Courage to Change

"Habit is stronger than reason," wrote philosopher George Santayana, and anyone with a verifiable bad habit is sure to agree. We can all probably think of a dozen good reasons why we shouldn't procrastinate so much, eat so much, and exercise so little. These reasons make sense, at least on an intellectual level. You probably can think of a dozen reasons why your habit is bad for you (and in the next chapter, we'll ask you to do just that).

But even having a clear understanding of the illogical and irrational nature of your habit doesn't automatically free you from its terrible hold. There's probably lots of stuff in your way, including a healthy dose of denial (see "It's Not Me, It's My Life", above), years of conditioned behavior, and a certain commitment to, if not love of, the habit itself.

To break through such obstacles takes courage, and finding that courage is an important step in the process of change. Start right now to think of the way your habit is undermining your goals, self-image, or relationships. Just by admitting the problem means that you've found at least some of the courage you'll need to break the habit that's been holding you back. Now go forward. You can do it!

The Least You Need to Know

➤ Habits are natural parts of everyday life.

➤ Any habit—even a healthy one—can turn bad.

➤ A bad habit undermines your sense of self-esteem, poses a danger to your health, and/or interferes in your personal or professional relationships.

➤ A stressful lifestyle can contribute to the development of a bad habit and become an obstacle to change.

➤ When a habit interferes with your life, it's time to break it.

➤ It takes courage and commitment to face and then, slowly but surely, to break a bad habit.

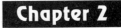

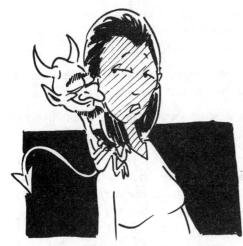

Why You Do the Things You Do

On Monday morning, your boss criticizes the report you spent the last three weekends preparing. By Friday, you've spent an entire week compulsively talking on the phone to friends, coworkers, anyone who would listen, about what you're going to do—except you haven't *really* done anything. Now your boss is steamed because the report's late *and* you've spent too much company time on personal calls.

Your children are demanding, your mother-in-law keeps nagging, and the washing machine breaks *again*. You'd think you'd be looking forward to a dinner out, but instead you're 45 minutes late—and not for the first time—to meet your husband, who sits fuming at the bar with his third glass of wine.

Bad habits. They're always there to fall back on. You feel let down at work, angry and frustrated at home, so you talk too much, you turn up late, you overeat...you find some way to release your negative feelings.

For a while, maybe even a long while, your bad habit appears to be a harmless distraction. But in the long run, your bad habit doesn't make your life any easier. (In fact, bad habits usually cause more problems than they solve, but we'll get to that later.)

So, now that you've flicked on this lightbulb of realization, you're probably eager to break your habit right away. You see the problem clearly, and now it's time to take action.

One Day at a Time

Separate your true self from your bad habit. Realize and accept that you're *not* your bad habit, nor are you a bad person for performing it. It's the habit that's the problem, not your personality, your integrity, or your will. By accepting this concept, you can avoid becoming stuck in a vicious cycle of low self-esteem, leading to failure, leading to even lower self-esteem.

You'll just stop. You're strong, you're proud. You're brave and true. You'll just say no.

And you will. But we have to break it to you: Kicking a bad habit is never an easy or short endeavor. Before you can do away with your bad habit for good, you're going to have to learn a little bit about *why* you developed it in the first place, and the role it now plays in your life.

We know what you're thinking. *"Why,"* you ask, *"can't I just stop? Why* do I need to know why I do something before I can stop doing it?" No process of change. No twelve, ten, or even two steps necessary. Just one. Starting now—no, maybe tomorrow—no more bad habit. *"Why not?"*

Well, try it and see. Chances are, you've *already* tried to stop it cold, and probably more than once. But when the pressure builds, your guard goes down, or the urge gets too great, you'll indulge your bad habit just a little bit. Then you'll indulge just a little bit more and a little bit more often, until before long, you're back in the grips of a full-fledged bad habit extravaganza. That's because you've never uncovered the root of the problem: the situations or feelings that trigger your bad habit in the first place.

"The only way round is through," wrote America's premier poet, Robert Frost. An elegant and beautiful way of saying that there's no easy way to solve a problem or learn a lesson, Frost's comment is particularly apt when it comes to the process involved in breaking bad habits. Plainly speaking, there's no easy way to let go of an ingrained behavior, no matter how much you want to or how damaging it is to your life. Instead, you've got to do some fairly serious self-examination beforehand to find out just why you do the things you do.

The Devil Made Me Do It

Do you remember your first time?

…The first time you and your habit become acquainted: your first drag of a cigarette, the first time you entered an online chat room, the first day (or week) of procrastination, the first knee-jiggle or unsuppressed belch?

Do you remember what it felt like? James remembers his very first cigarette, even though he smoked it more than 30 years ago at the age of 12. "At first it made me kind of nauseated, but then I also felt this rush. Part of it was the nicotine, I'm sure, but it was also all the other things that went with smoking: the danger (my mother would have skinned me alive had she caught me) and the 'coolness' of it. Also, my big brother was standing over me, waiting for me to choke so he could make fun of me. Even now, I know I also associate smoking with independence and being 'one of the guys.'"

For many people, the beginning of a bad habit starts out when they succumb to this compelling mixture of peer pressure, curiosity, danger, and excitement. For many people caught up in more severe addictions (i.e., alcoholism, drug abuse, serious gambling), their first time provides an actual physical "high"—one they forever strive, but never quite manage, to relive. Although the motivation is less intense for the average bad habit, there may be an element of this "search for past excitement" involved.

On the other hand, if you don't remember your first encounter with your bad habit, you're not alone. Many bad habits start out as benign behaviors hardly noticeable until they become so entrenched and distracting that they drive you (and sometimes everyone else, too) completely crazy. (Instead of an hour online, you're spending the whole evening—every evening!)

Now think about how you felt when you first became aware of your bad habit: Were you excited and stimulated by it at the start like James? Or did it kind of creep up on you?

In either case, the behavior most certainly didn't start out as a bad habit. You did it once, with either great fanfare or with almost no thought or intent at all. It only became a bad habit when you did it again, and then again and again—and you did that because, as senseless as drinking that fifth cup of coffee may seem now, your bad habit does indeed serve an important purpose in your life.

The Pleasure Principle

Now turn your thoughts to a more recent episode: Think about the very last time you performed your bad habit. What were you feeling just before you picked up that piece of Belgian chocolate, began a conversation with yourself on the street, or scrubbed your already immaculate bathroom floor? Check off all the emotions that apply—and be honest:

Column A	Column B
❏ Stressed out	❏ Relaxed
❏ Annoyed	❏ Satisfied
❏ Overwhelmed	❏ In control
❏ Bored	❏ Engaged
❏ Weak and/or unworthy	❏ Self-confident

Take a look at your answers. We'd be willing to bet that most of your choices fall into Column A, and very few, if any, into Column B. When you're feeling relaxed, in control, and self-confident, it's far less likely that you'll succumb to a behavior you know is ultimately damaging your health or well-being.

Instead, most people develop bad habits as a defense against *anxiety*, as a way to relieve the physical and emotional side effects of *stress*. And that's perfectly normal. In fact, relief or avoidance of anxiety is one of our species' most basic survival instincts.

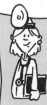

Strictly Speaking

Anxiety is a feeling of apprehension or uneasiness about an anticipated danger, whether real or imagined. **Stress** is the physical and emotional response to any demand—positive or negative—made upon a human being. The need to release feelings of anxiety and stress often leads to bad habits.

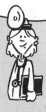

Strictly Speaking

Freud, the father or psychoanalysis, described the human mind as being divided between the **ego**, which is the conscious sense of self that experiences and maintains contact with reality, and the **id**, which is the part of the psyche working in the unconscious. Your ego may fully understand that a habit is doing you harm, but your id makes its own set of demands!

On May 6, 1856, a Viennese couple named Jakob and Amalie Freud gave birth to a baby boy they named Sigmund, who grew up to become one of the most influential thinkers of the twentieth century. In essence, Sigmund Freud invented modern psychiatry and psychoanalysis, and his theories forever changed our ideas about human behavior, emotion, thought, and motivation. Although currently under attack for their sex-biased and sex-obsessed aspects (to put a very simple spin on a complex argument), Freud's theories nonetheless still offer insight and perspective to many aspects of human behavior.

When it comes to understanding the role bad habits play in our lives, one of Freud's early ideas may be especially helpful. In 1911, he postulated that one of humankind's strongest drives is to avoid anxiety and pain—a theory he dubbed the *Pleasure Principle*. (Now you know where Janet Jackson got the name for that cool song.) Freud believed that in order to protect ourselves from anxiety, the *id*, the most primitive part of our unconscious, motivates us to take action against situations or emotions that challenge or threaten us.

One ineffective but relatively simple way we do that is by performing one (or two or three) of any number of actions that can, over time, become habits. And if those habits prevent us from meeting our goals or maintaining a secure sense of self, they're bad habits: They may relieve stress in the short term, but they also have negative side effects that crop up in the future.

What kind of situations triggers stress or anxiety? Do you even have to ask? Modern society is fraught with them. Even early in the twentieth century, before Elvis, fax machines, the Internet, Ab Crunchers, and reports of alien abduction, Freud recognized the challenges his fellow humans faced. He wrote: "Life as we find it is too hard for us; it entails too much pain, too many disappointments, impossible tasks. We cannot do without palliative [soothing, easing] remedies."

Practice Makes Perfect

"The chains of habit are too weak to be felt until they are too strong to be broken," wrote eighteenth-century writer-philosopher Samuel Johnson—and that statement certainly sums up how insidious the development of bad habits tends to be. Before you know it (even if it takes years), you're not just smoking one cigarette with an after dinner drink but chain-smoking ten cigarettes by mid-day. You don't just tell a fib or two to avoid hurting someone's feelings, you lie on a regular basis. Your credit card bills show that you don't just partake in a relatively harmless, occasional spending spree, but rather suffer from a buying fetish to rival the one enjoyed by Imelda Marcos.

Remember the "What's Your Lifestyle?" quiz you took in Chapter 1, "What Is a Bad Habit?" Well, if you have any questions about what triggers your bad habits, take another look at your results. Remember, the categories included:

➤ too much stress

➤ too little time

➤ boredom

➤ low self-esteem

What part of your life seems most out of control? Are you frustrated and overwhelmed by your work or personal responsibilities? Are you continually overscheduled? Do you feel unfulfilled and unmotivated? Could your ego use a little (or more than a little) boosting?

In later chapters, we'll help you identify your "bad habit triggers" with more specificity and accuracy. For now, it's important for you to understand that the urge to relieve stress or anxiety is a common denominator when it comes to the development of bad habits. Instead of dealing with the cause of anxiety in a straightforward way—standing up to your demanding boss or joining an exercise class—you *displace* or transfer your reaction from its source to another behavior.

> **Strictly Speaking**
> **Displacement** is the process or result of shifting an idea, activity, or emotional attachment from its proper object to another object. We all do it: The boss yells at us, but we take out our frustration not at her or at work, but at our cat or our lover or the wall. When it comes to bad habits, the act of smoking a cigarette instead of dealing with the fact you're bored or lonely is a form of displacement.

In short, bad habits serve to:

➤ relieve stress

➤ provide a "vacation" from a busy schedule

➤ distract you from boredom

➤ confirm your feelings of low self-esteem

The good news is that once you understand the nature of bad habits, and the role they play in alleviating the anxieties and stress in your life, you've begun to attack the problem at its root. As we'll explore further in later chapters, you have two basic options: You can reduce the source of anxiety triggering the bad habit, or you can transfer or displace your reaction to a healthier behavior (e.g., instead of binge eating when you're feeling anxious, you take a walk or do some yoga.

A New Angle

Although you can't exactly label them "habits," scientists have discovered that most if not all species of animals practice some kind of displacement: If a man approaches a mother bird nesting on her eggs, for instance, the bird will become quite agitated, not knowing whether to flee the impending danger or fight to protect her eggs. Instead of doing either, she begins to preen her feathers—a nervous reaction (and potential bad habit) if there ever was one!

When You Can't Give It Up

"But I don't think I'll be able to break my bad habit. I need it. I don't know what'll happen to me if I give it up."

That's what you're saying right now, isn't it? You're afraid that the inability to relieve stress through the normal route (i.e., your bad habit), you'll only end up feeling more anxious and upset than ever.

And you're right, at least at first. By its very nature change—even positive change—challenges your equilibrium, the relative balance you attempt to maintain every day. In other words, change causes stress, and as Freud just taught us, humans will do almost anything to avoid that ubiquitous but damaging internal and external force.

Among the most common reactions to, and defenses against, making changes are these:

➤ **Fear:** One of the strongest and most primal motivators of human behavior, fear is also the most common barrier to change. Fear of what it might be like to let go of a familiar habit as well as the fear of coming face to face with "the new you" (despite or perhaps because of the power, potential, and confidence you'll then embrace) can certainly hold you back from getting started.

➤ **Stubbornness:** Just plain stubbornness prevents many an individual burdened with a bad habit from moving forward. Take someone who—despite a weight problem and a heart condition—continues to eat red meat, buttered white bread, and sweets on a regular basis. "No one's going to tell me how to live my life," is the stubborn response of a person whose life is out of (not in!) control.

➤ **Self-destruction:** If your answers to the "What's Your Lifestyle?" quiz revealed that low self-esteem is a problem for you, your bad habits may be a direct or indirect method of punishing or hurting yourself. If the inability to hold your temper or remember important dates like birthdays or anniversaries interferes with your intimate relationships, for instance, your resistance to change could well mean that you feel unworthy of being loved or feeling secure.

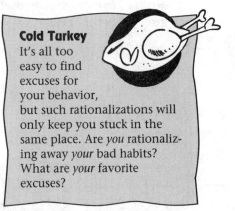

Cold Turkey
It's all too easy to find excuses for your behavior, but such rationalizations will only keep you stuck in the same place. Are *you* rationalizing away *your* bad habits? What are *your* favorite excuses?

➤ **Perfectionism:** Nothing is more undermining to the process of change than an unrealistic expectation of perfection. Perfectionists face challenges on many different fronts when it comes to bad habits: First, they have trouble admitting—to themselves and to others—that a problem exists. Second, perfectionists often procrastinate (compounding a bad habit) because they've got a terrible fear they'll fail, thus destroying their "perfect" image and ability to cope.

➤ **Fear of Failure/Learned Helplessness:** This obstacle often affects people who have tried and failed, and tried and failed again, to break their bad habits. In the annals of psychology, learned helplessness explains an interesting phenomenon: Mice (and presumably humans!) who have been unavoidably punished in the past will not act to avoid punishment later, even when avoidance is possible. Many people suffer a form of "learned helplessness" after trying again and again to break a bad habit. Their repeated failures cause them to simply give up instead of attempting another, potentially more successful, approach.

Considering all of these impressive stumbling blocks to change, it's remarkable that anyone manages to break a bad habit at all. But thousands of people do so every day, and so can you. You need to believe in yourself enough to follow a serious and informed plan, one that we'll help you create in Part 2.

Will the Real You Please Stand Up?

You're almost ready. You can feel it, can't you? You see that your bad habit amounts to nothing more than a passing distraction. You've begun to identify the situations and emotions that trigger your negative behavior. You recognize the stumbling blocks to success and look forward to finding ways to avoid or overcome them.

You're beginning to see the real you emerge from the shadow of your bad habit. Hold on to that positive image of yourself, and as you read on, it will soon become a vital and strong reality. Try this meditative exercise to reflect on becoming the person you want to be.

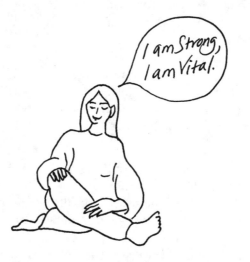

➤ Sit comfortably in a quiet room. Close your eyes. Take even, deep breaths. Let all the tension and stress flow from your body.

➤ When you've reached a calm state, begin to form a mental image of yourself as the strong, focused individual that you know you can be inside.

➤ Let go of your expectations of failure that you've learned in the past. If one should sneak past your strong defenses, banish it immediately with your next deep breath.

➤ Now, imagine within yourself a wellspring of strength and power. It may be in your abdomen, at the center of your forehead, even in the palm of your hand. Draw from that well-spring whenever you feel your self-confidence begin to flag.

Now that you've started to sort out why you do the things you do, we're ready to outline a variety of bad habits—one or more of which may plague you. In the next chapter, we discuss cravings (for substances such as nicotine, caffeine, and sugar), tendencies (to indulge in behaviors like procrastination to lying to losing one's temper), and compulsions (to clean, shop, gamble, and undermine relationships). Although by nature habits have many similarities, each bad habit has its own set of unique qualities that you'll need to explore before you can rid yourself of it.

The Least You Need to Know

➤ Bad habits form as reactions to stressful events.

➤ Avoidance of stress is a normal human drive.

➤ Resistance to change is natural, but can be overcome.

➤ Defenses against changing bad habits include fear, stubbornness, self-destructive behavior, perfectionism, and feelings of helplessness.

➤ Separating who you are from your bad habits helps you think positively and welcome change.

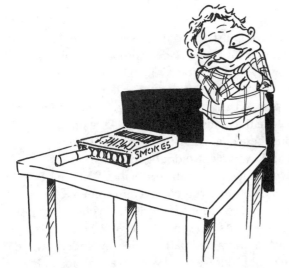

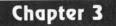

But I Like It Like That

Believe it or not: The process you'll use to break a habit is almost identical no matter what habit has you in its grips. You'll use the same basic strategies to quit belching with abandon in public, twirling strands of hair round and round (and round) your index finger, or "forgetting" to hang up your clothes at the end of the day.

That said, we believe it may be helpful to briefly explore the dynamics of specific categories of habits and the "attractions" each category offers. Indeed, all habits are not alike, and you may discover something about what motivates your particular vice by reading about these bad habit categories.

Go Figure

No one knows exactly why one person cleans compulsively to relieve anxiety while another smokes cigarettes and still another procrastinates. Accident probably explains some of it: The first time you start to feel oogy, your knee starts to jiggle. It works to relieve your ooginess, and so you do it again and again until, sooner or later, it drives everyone else insane! Genetics likely play a part in this, as in everything, although I don't imagine that scientists will ever isolate the gene that causes knuckle-cracking or belching in public (which would allow us to breed out these characteristics). The most likely culprits are the old standbys: environment and example. No doubt you once witnessed behavior that formed your current bad habit. You might be mimicking similar conduct you observed in someone close to you or, conversely, reacting against it (i.e., you eat too fast because your brother eats too slowly). At some point, this behavior became an ingrained part of your life. Indeed, there seems to be no doubt that we learn how to act by absorbing the behavior of others around us.

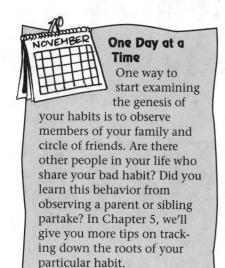

One Day at a Time

One way to start examining the genesis of your habits is to observe members of your family and circle of friends. Are there other people in your life who share your bad habit? Did you learn this behavior from observing a parent or sibling partake? In Chapter 5, we'll give you more tips on tracking down the roots of your particular habit.

When we started researching this book, we discovered an interesting project established by the Centers for Disease Control in Atlanta. Called the Behaviorial Risk Factor Surveillance System (sounds like something Scully and Mulder might use on *The X-Files*, doesn't it?), this survey regularly gathers information about the health habits of the average American, state by state. We're still waiting for the complete results (ah, government agencies), but the highlights of the latest report released on July 31, 1997 showed these interesting facts:

➤ The highest percentage (22.9 percent) of *binge drinkers* (defined as those who imbibe more than 5 drinks at a sitting) live in Wisconsin, perhaps not so surprising since Milwaukee remains the beer-brewing capital of the United States. What is strange, however, is that the lowest percentage (5.2) of binge drinkers live in Tennessee, a state that offers up the finest bourbons in the world.

➤ The highest percentage of *couch potatoes* (48.6) live in—are you sitting down?—Washington, D.C., which explains a *lot* when you think about it. Colorado might feel quite uncomfortable to those of us who have trouble with our "get up and go": 73.8 percent of Coloradans exercise on a regular basis.

➤ The highest percentage of *smokers* (22.8) live in Kentucky, which makes sense since more tobacco grows there than anywhere else in the nation. Utah has the lowest percentage (13.2), perhaps because so many Mormons—who are prohibited by religious tenet to use tobacco—live in and around Salt Lake City.

➤ The highest percentage of *seat-belt wearers* (86.9) live in Hawaii, and the lowest (41.4 percent) live in North Dakota. We have absolutely no idea what this indicates about either the states or the people who live in them. Interesting, though, isn't it?

It really is too bad that no government agency has yet to conduct surveys on other common bad habits. Wouldn't it be great to know where the most liars live? Or what state to avoid if you can't stand messy living rooms? Or where to move if your family has banished you and your gum-snapping ways? But we are individuals, not statistics, right? So we must look at bad habits—even ones that have a known state bias—as very personal issues with quite individual motivations.

What Kind of Idiot Are You?

How do you react to anxiety? What's your remedy for stress, overscheduling, boredom, or feelings of low self-esteem? The answers to the following questions may help you figure that out.

1. Your date cancels plans for Saturday night at the last minute. Do you:

   (a) Take a swig of brandy straight from the bottle.

   (b) Tell all your friends you're actually in Paris for the weekend.

   (c) Feel compelled to turn on a cable TV shopping channel with credit card in hand.

2. A huge project comes up at work and you're on deadline to finish it. Your first instinct is to:

   (a) Chain smoke like there's no tomorrow.

   (b) Watch a movie (or a triple feature) until you feel more "motivated."

   (c) Bet your coworker $50 that you'll finish on time.

3. You've just found out you're spending the holidays with your spouse's entire family. The first thing you want to do is:

   (a) Brew your fifth cup (or pot) of coffee.

   (b) "Forget" to pick up the kids from day care.

   (c) Clean your already immaculate bathroom, again.

4. Something's on your mind, but you're not sure what's bothering you. You:

    (a) Cook (and consume) Thanksgiving dinner—in June.

    (b) Hope that whatever it is, it takes care of itself. And snap at anyone who tries to get you to focus on any kind of problem whatsoever.

    (c) Spend $100 calling 900 numbers from hot lines that predict the future.

5. You finally made it to a friend's party, where you're determined to meet someone new. As you try to mingle, you:

    (a) Offer to pass the hors d'oeuvres as a way to start conversations but end up using the tasty tray of treats as a ploy to eat a lot without anyone noticing.

    (b) Actually, you lost the directions to the party and just couldn't make it! Maybe next time...

    (c) Wash your hands 17 times to make sure you're presentable.

6. You finally purchased your gym membership. You've made a solemn promise to work out three times a week. When it's time for your first weight-training class, you:

    (a) Decide to finish your "last" pack of cigarettes, since quitting smoking is definitely a part of your health kick.

    (b) Feel terrible because that *absolutely essential* telephone call at the office made you too late for class, so you walk the treadmill for five minutes and go home.

    (c) Decide not to go because your workout clothes aren't perfectly spotless and you know you just won't have the same kind of energy if you're not perfectly clad! Not you!

How many *A*'s did you score? *B's? C's?* The answers may tell you something about your natural, instinctive response to stress:

A—Cravings. If you've checked off more than a few *A*'s, your instinct tells you to go for the substance, whether it's alcohol, nicotine, caffeine, or food, when you feel stress or anxiety.

B—Tendencies. If you've checked off lots of *B*'s, you've learned to avoid dealing with difficult situations by losing your temper, "forgetting" about it, or telling a lie (to yourself or to others). In other words, you've become pretty good at displacing your frustration and anxiety not with substances or direct activities, but by undermining your relationships. You may also be terrific at avoiding a problem altogether, by simply procrastinating.

C—Compulsions. A preponderance of *C* answers tells you that when you feel anxious or under stress, you need to *act*, to *do* something to relieve those uncomfortable feelings. You tap your feet, twirl your hair, or grind your teeth. Or you vent your anxiety by indulging in that one person, place, or thing you just can't get enough of.

What do you think? Does your bad habit fall into one of these categories? We identified these bad habit categories—cravings, tendencies, and compulsions—by first listing every bad habit we could think of (or at least the most common ones), and then contrasting and comparing their individual characteristics. Do understand, though, that these categories are not based on strict, medical definitions and may overlap with one another.

Constant Cravings

We've all experienced one or two of them—a lust for chocolate, a yearning for french fries, a *need* for nicotine. Although you can also crave solitude or excitement, we relate the word "cravings" to substances that you eat, drink, or inhale. In Part 3, we'll be discussing the bad habits that can develop when you satisfy these cravings—despite their potential health risks—instead of facing life's ups and downs head on.

➤ **Alcohol.** To drink or not to drink, that is the question. Alcohol is an integral part of our culture, especially at certain times and places in our lives. Many people develop a problem with alcohol in college, for instance, where drinking becomes the ultimate release from social and academic pressures.

➤ **Cigarettes.** There is no reason in the world to start smoking and every reason in the world to stop. So why do more than 40 million Americans still light up on a regular basis? Probably because nicotine is one of the most addictive substances known to man or woman, and a little experimentation in adolescence can lead to a life-long habit.

A New Angle

We all know that smoking causes innumerable health problems, but this plain and simple fact may help support your commitment to breaking your nicotine habit: The average healthy 35-year-old man cuts 7.1 years off his life expectancy by smoking. And women smokers have just as much to worry about: Their risk for lung cancer has more than quadrupled since 1964, and is greater than the risk of breast cancer!

➤ **Caffeine.** The smell (and taste) of coffee in the morning is such a common craving that scientists who study body rhythms refer to it as a Zeitgeber, or "time-giver." There are few among us who don't depend on the jolt a cup or two of coffee (or other caffeinated beverage) gives us to get us up and running. Unfortunately, a dependency on caffeine can become very disruptive, both physically and emotionally.

➤ **Food.** Who ever would have thought that the basic human need for nutrition would become so laden with psychological, physical, and—for many people—pathological aspects? People don't eat just to satisfy hunger. They also eat because they're bored, depressed, angry, or lonely. And pleasure and satisfaction aren't always the result of eating. Instead, eating (especially uncontrolled eating) triggers feelings of low self-esteem and depression as well.

Tempting Tendencies

"Easier said than done." Many people take this saying far too literally. Instead of facing up to the complexity of relationships or the complications of life in general, they rely on emotional outbursts to distract them. Another all too common tendency is to procrastinate, or put off dealing with a challenge altogether. You'll find out more about tempting tendencies—and how to overcome them—in Part 4, but here are a couple of examples:

Strictly Speaking
Passive aggression means acting out strong feelings or opinions in an indirect manner. Although it's usually used to describe a relationship dynamic, you can also be passive aggressive with yourself. Missing a deadline or wallowing in disorganization can be ways of indirectly expressing feelings of low self-esteem or self-loathing.

➤ **Poor Communication.** Flying off the handle, "forgetting" (a passive-aggressive behavior if there ever was one), undermining: there are any number of ways to do it: Lying is a biggie, so is losing your temper, forgetting, simply not participating in an open and honest way. All of these tendencies help you avoid what's really going on in the relationship.

➤ **Procrastination.** Do you have any idea how long Suzanne put off writing this paragraph? No kidding. Writing about procrastination hits too close to home, and so she tried to avoid doing it at all—a typical response. When she talked to Gary about it, he revealed his own secret: He too procrastinates, and usually does so when the task at hand involves an uncomfortable emotion. Ironically enough, however, he sometimes procrastinates by writing, an activity that allows him to distance himself from that emotion.

Compelling Compulsions

Compulsion was a terrific movie made by Orson Welles in 1965. Based on the true story of a famous legal case known as Leopold and Loeb, the movie depicted the drive to murder that the two rich boys felt, and the terrible act this compulsion "forced" them to commit. Most compulsions involve far less pathological activities, but the drive to perform them is often just as strong. You'll find out more about them in Part 5, but here are a few examples:

➤ **Fidgeting.** Gum-snapping, hair-twirling, knee-jiggling, toe-tapping…these are just a few of the fidgeting behaviors that help to release the very real physical symptoms of stress and tension. Most of the time, the first people to recognize these bad habits are those who have to witness them—friends, lovers, business associates—who slowly but surely are driven to distraction by your incessant movement.

➤ **Personal Release.** Okay. This is one of Suzanne's pet peeves. Brought up in a small New England town where manners were valued above most other human qualities, she's never understood the freedom some others feel to release pent-up gasses by belching or passing wind in public. In other cultures, such biological emissions are signs of a deep appreciation of a hearty meal (in the case of belching) or merely an unavoidable side effect of digestion. Here in the States, however, intentional personal releases remain unseemly and unpleasant to most people.

➤ **Compulsive Cleaning.** Some people deal with anxiety and stress by bringing the adage "cleanliness is next to godliness" to a literal quest for perfection, order, and control over their environment. Constant scrubbing, endless straightening, or perpetual prissiness certainly redirects one's energy—energy that might be better spent on coping with what really needs to be straightened out.

➤ **Sloppiness.** Can't file your taxes because you've lost your receipts in a pile of paper the size and complexity of the Great Sphinx? Unable to attend the "get-to-know-you" neighborhood party because every article of clothing you own is in the laundry (or stuffed into the bottom of the closet)? When you think about it, sloppiness sure does provide some good, if unhealthy, excuses for avoiding certain challenges. It can also be a passive-aggressive way to express anger or feelings of low self-esteem.

➤ **Financial Chaos.** Money troubles. Who doesn't have one or two in this era of high expectations and only average paychecks? However, chronic

Cold Turkey
Warning! Avoid judging yourself by the bad habits you indulge in or the good habits you neglect. Once you start down that path, you may never see the light of day. Instead, reassess your goals and the means you have to achieve them, emphasize your assets, and move forward.

problems with money—including overspending, neglecting bills and taxes, and gambling—usually indicate some bad financial habits, probably motivated by the feelings of unrelieved stress, pressure, boredom, and low self-esteem.

Do you see your bad habit in any of these three general categories? Do you have more than one bad habit falling into more than one category? Some people's bad habits seem to pile up and eventually cross over. How about the person who relieves marital stress by having lots of affairs (see "Compelling Compulsions"), then lies quite seamlessly about them, (see "Tempting Tendencies"), and to top it off, frequently drinks too much alcohol (no doubt to relieve guilt, another common source of stress—see "Constant Cravings"). One bad habit really *can* lead to another.

Striving for Balance

In the *Random House Dictionary*, one definition of the word balance is "a state of stability, as of the body or the emotions"; another refers to balance as "a state of harmony." Without question, stability and harmony are two important keys to emotional, physical, and psychological good health.

And one sure-fire way to throw yourself off balance is to develop a really entrenched bad habit. Cigarette smoking, for example, most directly affects the health of your lungs and your cardiovascular system; it also may prevent you from exercising on a regular basis or enjoying the taste of your food (leading to bad eating habits). It may even trigger sloppy housekeeping habits (why clean the kitchen when ashes and the smell of smoke will mar the atmosphere before long?). We'll talk more about bad habit complications in Part 2.

Without sounding too "New Agey," restoring balance and harmony to your life is one of the major goals and benefits of breaking your bad habit. Stop smoking and you'll probably want to start exercising and eating right—and not only because you'll have rejuvenated your heart and taste buds, but also because of the important boost you'll give to your self-esteem and the sense of commitment to yourself and to your goals.

New Year's Resolutions

Let's get it straight right from the start. When it comes to breaking bad habits, every day has the potential to be New Year's Day—the day you start your new, bad-habit–free life. There's absolutely no reason for you to wait until January 1.

On the other hand, one of the most common mistakes when it comes to breaking bad habits is believing the "No time like the present" and "Just do it" myths. Such a get-up-and-go attitude sounds positive and empowering, but it also has a downside: Trying to do too much—or expect too much, too soon—can really backfire.

What you can start right now is the *process of change*. You can begin to learn about the physical, psychological, and emotional adjustments breaking a bad habit requires you to make. If you take the time to follow through on a well-developed plan, you're more likely to be successful—in the short term and in the long term.

The Least You Need to Know

➤ Bad habits often fall into three categories: cravings, tendencies, and compulsions.

➤ In addition to looking inside yourself, look at the people around you and the environment you live in for clues about the origins of your nasty habits.

➤ No matter what your bad habit is, you'll use the same behavioral techniques to break it.

➤ Breaking a bad habit is a *process*, not a decision. Deciding to shoot your albatross is only one step on the road to freedom from a habit that is doing you no good.

Part 2
Just Say No!

You know you want to change, but you've tried before and it didn't work. At the most, you might make it three weeks without your bad habit sneaking back into your life.

What it takes to really break your bad habit is one part self-examination, two parts determination, and three parts tenacity. You'll need to:

➤ *Identify your bad habit and the forms it takes.*

➤ *Weigh the positive and negative aspects of your bad habit.*

➤ *Discover healthy substitutes and sources of motivation.*

➤ *Recognize the potential for relapse and prepare for it.*

➤ *Imagine the new, habit-free you and go for it!*

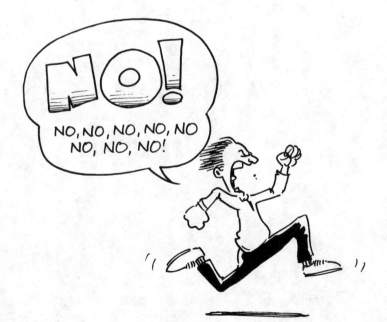

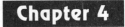

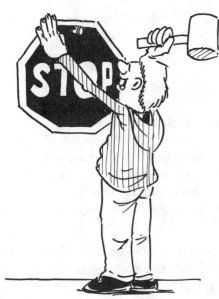

Okay, So How Do You Stop?

Get ready, get set... GO! You're in your way. Oops, we mean, you're ON your way. Wow, look at what just happened. A universal truth about bad habits has revealed itself in all its Freudian slip glory! Your bad habits, the habits you clutch to yourself like a warm overcoat on a blustery day, are the very behaviors that could be forming a barrier between you and the fulfillment and enjoyment of your deepest personal dreams, aspirations, and desires.

It comes down to a matter of priorities: Which do you love more—your goals (The frightening but exhilarating things you'd like to do. Anything from backpacking through Nepal with a Sherpa guide to playing a really serious game of golf...), or the bad habits that keep you chained to the same old, same old? ("Nepal?" you say, "I can't get off the couch. I guess it's the Discovery channel for me. Besides, I can't hike that far; I'm not in shape and I need to lose weight. Did you microwave that cheese popcorn for me?" Or, "I'll never be able to concentrate enough and relax into a good golf state of mind. Got any more coffee?") Sir Walter Scott said it best back at the start of the nineteenth century,

"Oh what a tangled web we weave, When first we practice to deceive!" But it turns out, we're only kidding ourselves. To break a bad habit, you have to learn how to get out of your own way.

Rome Wasn't Built in a Day

Well, you've been wrapping that coat of bad habits pretty tightly around your body for a long time. It worked nicely for you during the hard winter, didn't it? But guess what? Summer's coming. Every day gets a little bit warmer and that coat isn't so comfortable any more. You want to take it off but you just aren't quite sure you won't need it again. So you waver between the *familiar* discomfort of your bad habits and the *unfamiliar* discomfort of life without them. You come up with amazing, ingenious strategies to wear the bad habit coat even in 90-degree heat...lemonade on ice, anyone?

Well, Rome wasn't built in a day. Change is hard. It takes significant effort, commitment, and time to effect significant change. Failing to recognize that truth is what gets most people into trouble as they attempt to break their bad habits. They'd rather spend their effort preserving the habit; it *seems* easier—even if it's really not easier.

The thing is, most modern Americans have grown up believing that everything is supposed to be easy. Zap food in the microwave and dinner's ready in five minutes or less. All manner of human tragedy and frailty is resolved in under sixty minutes during our favorite sitcoms and dramas. Thin thighs in thirty days, seven days to a better you—it's hard not to believe that whatever needs doing can be done with practically the snap of your fingers.

Unfortunately, that's not the way it works. Life is messy, human nature is stubborn, and time—not efficiency—really *is* the great healer. In your heart, you probably know that already. So let's find out how to take off that bad habit coat for good. Jettison the coat; you don't need it any more. It's time to take a walk in the sunshine. What's that Zen saying about a long journey begins with a single step?

Learning to Live With or Without It: The Biology of Habit

On a purely physiological level, human beings appear to be remarkably adaptable creatures. Jump into a pool of cold water and, within a few uncomfortable, freezing moments, you actually begin to feel refreshed. Your body adapts, regulating body temperature, heart rate, and respiration to meet the change in the environment. This process is known as *homeostasis*.

This ability to adjust to often dramatic changes in our environment is what allows us to survive as a species. However, when you think about it, homeostasis is *not* about change, but rather about stability, about maintaining the same internal environment no matter what's happening on the outside.

Biologically speaking, that's the way we like it—just the same as always—and the body will work overtime if necessary to maintain its internal equilibrium. Blood sugar and blood pressure rise and fall in reaction to internal or external changes in the environment (say, eating a doughnut or arguing with a teenager), allowing the body to continue to function in as normal and stable a way as possible. We eat, we run, we get scared, we fall in love and our internal environment remains pretty stable over the long haul.

Homeostasis applies to our psychological life as well. New information enters through our senses and makes its way to the brain, which then breaks it down and integrates it into the established emotional and intellectual structure—making whatever adjustments are necessary. In most cases, the adjustments are minor and easily accommodated. When the newsstand doesn't have *The Wall Street Journal* one morning, we feel a pang of disappointment, but quickly rearrange our expectations and settle for *The New York Times*.

However, if the information threatens us in a fundamental way—the news of an unexpected death of a loved one or other trauma, for example—we have several defense mechanisms to protect us. Denial is a perfect example of such a defense. We do not acknowledge the information right away, but instead filter it slowly to give our minds and bodies time to adjust. Without such a defense, we'd be far too vulnerable to potentially damaging disruption.

You can see how hard you work to maintain a sense of "normalcy." You do it, in part, by relying on familiar thought and behavior patterns you've learned over time. It's easy to walk down a flight of stairs. You don't think about picking up your foot or negotiating the distance between each stair with every step you take. If you did, your body and mind would be in a state of constant overload. (Watch a small child's effort of physical and mental concentration to see what we mean.) Instead, you learned how to go up and down steps in a very deep and natural way a long time ago. Now, the activity is automatic.

And so it is with habits, good and bad. Your body learns that right after you brush your teeth, you rinse your mouth with water from the glass that sits to the right of the faucet. Pretty soon, your hand simply goes for the glass, without you having to "tell" it to go there with a conscious thought.

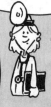

As a child, Suzanne remembers watching as her mother picked up and lit a cigarette as soon as the telephone rang, then smoked away during the conversation. Gary, ever the psychologist, asserts this wasn't a display of purely Pavlovian instinct or *conditioned reflex*; it wasn't exactly the sound of the bell that triggered a craving for nicotine. Instead, over the years, having a smoke while she chatted had become an ingrained behavior. It would have felt uncomfortable—unnatural even—without the cigarette in her hand, to say nothing of the nicotine coursing through her veins.

Habits become almost automatic *reflexes* that your body expects to perform under certain circumstances. They slowly but surely become part of your repertoire of behavior without you ever making the conscious decision to include them in your life.

Now it feels "normal" for you to bite your nails when you feel under a bit of stress because your body learned that behavior many years ago. If you don't bite your nails—if you consciously break the pattern—your body and mind will rebel. You'll probably feel uncomfortable, both physically and emotionally—at least until *not* biting your nails becomes the habit your body best remembers.

The biology of bad habits really comes into play when the habit involves substances—alcohol, nicotine, fat, sugar, caffeine, to name the most common culprits. These substances act to change brain and body chemistry in a much more direct way than other learned behaviors. Not only does the act of picking up a drink become a natural, learned reaction to stress, but the feelings that the alcohol itself trigger are also addictive.

We hope you now have a deeper understanding of how habits become so ingrained, and why breaking them is so difficult. The fact is, you have to "unlearn" the behavior that has become second nature to you. You can do so either by breaking the chain of events that leads to it in the first place, or by learning a new response to the same triggers. When you do this successfully, you'll finally be able to maintain a healthy internal physical and psychological environment, and the balance and harmony we first discussed in Chapter 3, "But I Like It Like That," will become the natural state your body craves.

"But wait," you say. "I'm not ready. My homeostasis is fine just the way it is, thank you. That bad habit isn't a really baaaaaaaad one. I don't need to unlearn it. Not yet. Maybe tomorrow. There's always tomorrow."

Well, we've heard that one before.

The Scarlett O'Hara Syndrome, or "I'll Think About It Tomorrow"

"I can't think about that today. I'll think about it tomorrow. After all, tomorrow is another day."

Remember those lines? (Sipping a Mint Julep might help bring back the memory.) A Southern belle named Scarlett O'Hara uttered them many times during *Gone with the Wind*, the 1939 best-seller and epic Academy Award-winning movie. The most memorable utterance occurred at the very end of the movie, when Rhett Butler, the love of her life, had had his fill of Scarlett's very bad habits and left her bereft on Tara's front staircase.

Without a doubt, Scarlett was her own worst enemy. Talk about a person with some bad habits! Let's take a look at some of Scarlett's most glaring undermining proclivities.

> ➤ **Cravings:** Food and Drink. Scarlett makes some bad decisions based on an obsession with an 18-inch waist, reinforced by Mammy who always seemed willing to cinch the corset stays that strangling inch tighter. And don't forget Scarlett's fondness for brandy.

> ➤ **Tendencies:** To lie. Big time—about everything. And of course, to procrastinate. What's that about tomorrow?

> ➤ **Compulsions:** Fidgeting. "Oh Fiddle-dee-dee," she'd say, as her toe tapped madly with impatience. Lusting after other women's husbands—a potential sexual addiction if there ever was one!

Cold Turkey
We mentioned it first in Chapter 1, but it bears repeating here: Serious addiction often requires professional medical and psychological attention. If you feel that your habit is out-of-control and threatening your health and welfare in a significant way, please discuss the matter with a licensed health care professional right away.

Although Scarlett O'Hara remains a worthy symbol of independence and spunk, her bad habits didn't really do her any good service. And we can all use this lesson Scarlett never managed to learn: Waiting for tomorrow doesn't justify the shenanigans we may be up to today. Procrastination and denial can put us up against a wall of ugly desperation. Face it, would you want to be reduced to making a dress out of draperies? Probably not.

However, before you start beating yourself up (again) about your own bad habits, there are, in fact, at least two legitimate reasons to wait another day (or month) before beginning the process of change:

➤ **It's not such a bad habit.** Be careful about pulling this rabbit out of the hat. Sure, one espresso a day might not be so bad, but three, well…. In the next chapter, we'll talk about establishing a "Daily Habit Log." Observe your habit with the detachment of a stranger and consider whether you're better off with or without it.

➤ **It's a terrible time.** If you're currently under a great deal of pressure or stress—if you're in the middle of a divorce, getting ready to move, changing jobs, or dealing with an illness—you may feel this isn't the optimal time for you to work on breaking your bad habit. Give yourself some slack; set some goals for the future, including breaking your bad habits, and stick to them.

But the most common reason people put off starting the process of change, however, is not because they feel it's truly unnecessary or that other pressures are just too great. It's not even because they're too lazy. It's because they're too afraid.

Facing Your Fears

You've been living with your bad habit for awhile now, and it's probably very difficult for you to imagine a time when you won't depend on it to get you through your day. You're afraid you simply won't be able to cope.

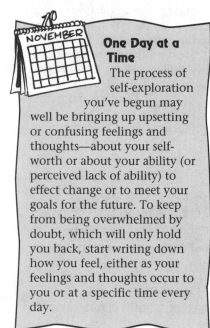

One Day at a Time
The process of self-exploration you've begun may well be bringing up upsetting or confusing feelings and thoughts—about your self-worth or about your ability (or perceived lack of ability) to effect change or to meet your goals for the future. To keep from being overwhelmed by doubt, which will only hold you back, start writing down how you feel, either as your feelings and thoughts occur to you or at a specific time every day.

This reaction is perfectly normal. After all, you count on your bad habit to simply maintain the biological and psychological status quo that includes your habit.

More than likely, however, one of your greatest fears is the fear of failure. Chances are, you've been here before, maybe more than once. You thought, then, that it would be a relative snap to turn off the television instead of watching all day and night, or cut down on your compulsive cleaning, stop fidgeting during important meetings. You just said no, and stopped—for one day, maybe two, maybe more.

But then you started again. And when you did, you felt crummy, worthless, weak, and ridiculous. You felt ashamed or frustrated that your own drama (or sitcom!) didn't resolve itself in 30 or 60 minutes, or just a week or two of trouble. Maybe you've repeated this cycle more than once until now you just might prefer living with the negative effects of your bad habit rather than face that failure even one more time.

Let it go. Right now. Today is a new day. This time will be different than all the others because you'll have all the information you need right at your fingertips. Already, you probably understand better than ever before that your bad habit isn't a mysterious curse visited upon you from above, or a sign of a terrible flaw in your character. Instead, you now know that it is merely a learned behavior your body's become accustomed to—and that you have the power and strength to unlearn that behavior if you give yourself the time and tools necessary.

Erasing the Tape

An undermining adage if there ever was one, "one step forward and two steps back" nevertheless sums up the experience of many a bad habit-breaker, especially at the start. Just when you think you're ready to change your behavior, just when you've made that first important move—admitting the problem and the desire to change—something gets in the way. That something is YOU!! (We've come full circle now.) More often than not, you're your own worst enemy. The negative emotions you have about yourself and about your history of missed opportunities (at least in the area of breaking bad habits) may well be the greatest barriers to success you'll face.

You hear it inside your head, don't you? That little voice (your own, your parent's, your first grade teacher's) that tells you that you'll never succeed, not this time, not ever. The little voice that uses words and phrases to undermine instead of support, judge instead of challenge, frustrate instead of encourage.

A New Angle

Recent studies show that what you do and what you think changes your body and brain chemistry. For instances, we know that when faced with a stressful situation or thought, your blood pressure goes up and certain areas in the brain become hyperactive. And the reverse is true: Pleasant thoughts activate a part of the brain that triggers feelings of satisfaction, and deep, relaxing breathing brings down blood pressure and heart rate. If you incorporate positive thinking and relaxation techniques into your lifestyle, you'll create an internal environment more conducive to change.

Before you can get down to the dirty work of breaking your habit, you need to erase any negative messages left on this "internal tape" or it's unlikely you'll find the courage or the strength to make the change.

Listen carefully to what you tell yourself and, even if you don't really mean it at first, change the vocabulary you use. Here are just a few suggestions to get you started:

Change...	To...
I'm a failure.	I've failed at some tasks in the past.
I shouldn't do that.	I prefer not to do that.
I must change.	I want to change.
I'm a bad person.	My behavior is undesirable.

Change all of your "I shoulds" and "I musts" to "I want tos" and "I prefer tos." By doing so, you'll put yourself back in the driver's seat; you'll be the one in control of your behavior and the changes you choose to make. We often don't pay any attention to the thoughts that parade through our minds on any given day; we don't question or examine them. Start doing this today. Recast negative judgments and feelings with more positive goals and emotions.

Take One Step Forward

Are you ready? Of course you are. In the chapters that follow, we'll take you through the process of change, step by step. You may want to read through all four of them first, and then go back and follow through on the suggestions that appeal to you. On the other hand, you may decide to take the bull by the horns and tackle each step as it comes. See what you think—whatever works for you is the right way. In the meantime, here's a brief overview of what's to come as you make the journey from bad habit to balance and harmony:

➤ **Identify the behavior.** You can't break a habit unless you know when and why you perform it. Chapter 5, "Step 1: Identify the Behavior," offers you a number of tips to help you track down your triggers and terrors.

➤ **Evaluate the risks and benefits.** Clearly, your bad habit has both positive and negative appeal. It offers you pleasure or relieves your stress (the positive), which is why you've held on to it for so long. It also holds you back or undermines your health in some way (the negative), which is why you're excited about breaking it. Chapter 6, "Step 2: Evaluate the Risks and Benefits," will help you understand the push-and-pull nature of bad habits—and realistically set the balance in favor of change.

➤ **Prepare for Change.** Look around. Do you still have a pack of cigarettes in the drawer? (How can you expect to stop if you do?) Is your jaw locked tight from grinding your teeth? (Wouldn't a massage or a yoga class feel good?) Are you alone on this journey? (Think of how helpful a support system might be when times get tough.) In Chapter 7, "Step 3: Prepare for Change," we'll help you create an environment conducive to the changes you want to make in your life and help you remove temptation and stress.

➤ **Just Do It.** By the time you make it to Chapter 8, "Step 4: Just Do It!" you're ready for action, and we'll show you the many techniques available, including physical substitutions, spiritual aids, and positive lifestyle changes.

How do you feel now? Nervous? Reassured? Afraid that you'll fail? (Don't worry. Even if you do "fail" by relapsing, you'll still be ahead of the game—and we'll show you how to get right back on track in Chapter 9, "Get Back on That Horse.") Excited??? We hope so. Now take a deep breath, you're on your way!

The Least You Need to Know

➤ Habits, good and bad, change our body chemistry.

➤ Just as you can learn a bad habit, you can unlearn it.

➤ Getting out of your own way and letting go of your fear are the first things that have to happen before you can start in on breaking your bad habit.

➤ It's important to replace negative messages with positive self-talk.

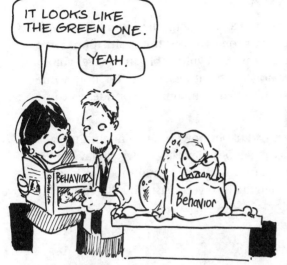

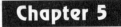

Chapter 5

Step 1: Identify the Behavior

In This Chapter

➤ Getting to the root of your bad habit

➤ Tracking your bad habit through the day

➤ Identifying your bad habit triggers

➤ Taking control of the controls

"Deep experience is never peaceful," American author Henry James once wrote. Now that you're starting to really contemplate your bad habit and how it affects your life, we bet you know just what he means. It isn't easy facing your demon of choice because that means taking a pretty close look at yourself and your inner motivations.

Whether it's something relatively benign like having to eat every meal from your favorite plate or a behavior with potential health consequences like consuming a high-fat, low nutrient diet, the bad habit you have developed is a response to some uncomfortable inner truth or early training. You've become accustomed to the feeling that performing your habit gives you and, to some degree, you depend on the habit to get you through the day.

Who, Where, When, Why, How?

We're going to ask you take stock of your habit in a very methodical and honest way. What you'll be looking for is quite specific: The people, places, times, situations, or emotions (during the day or in your life) that leave you vulnerable and trigger you to perform your bad habit. You'll also explore how the habit makes you feel, both while you're performing it and then later, when you've had some time to consider its consequences.

Before you look at the here and now of your bad habit, however, you might find it helpful to uncover some of its deeper roots (remember Alex Haley—we all have roots!), especially if your bad habit is one that's developed over time in adulthood or is something you've done since you were little. By delving into your past, you'll no doubt discover some clues to your present behavior.

Uprooting Your Bad Habit(s)

Most habits have some very deep and complex roots. Taking a look at those roots and tracing them to their source may yield surprising and unexpected information about who you are. That's what happened for Amy, one of Gary's former clients.

At 34, Amy's been overweight for much of her adult life. She's tried all sorts of diets, fasts, and exercise plans, but nothing seems to work. Before she knows it, she's eating too much of the wrong kinds of food and gaining weight all over again. "I lack willpower" is the reason she offers for her lack of success, and inside she thinks "I'm weak" and "I'm worthless." She has no clue that there may be other reasons why she can't seem to lose weight no matter how hard she tries.

Through her sessions with Gary, Amy talked about her family relationships, and by doing so, shed some light on her own relationship to food.

It turns out that Amy's mother, Clara, grew up during the Great Depression, as did many of our parents. Amy's grandfather got by as a day laborer on other people's farms and her grandmother took in sewing. Sometimes Clara's family ate three meals a day, and sometimes they went hungry. So as a child, Amy's mom learned to associate a full stomach with a feeling of well-being, security, and love.

The family struggled, but Clara went on to become a successful lawyer married to a corporate executive. She cooked elaborate family meals and enjoyed the feeling of carrying an extra few pounds.

As soon as Amy was born, feeding her daughter became Clara's way of showing love. Clara told her daughter what it was like to be poor, and made Amy feel fearful that they too could be poor someday. Then, as Amy got older, her mother made her feel guilty for not eating the rich, gourmet foods she cooked. Clara worked long hours at times, and she would leave behind desserts for Amy to eat when she got home from school, along with a note telling her how much she loved her.

By the time she reached her 20s, Amy had developed quite an entrenched weight problem. It got worse when she moved to a big city and started her career. Overwhelmed, Amy found herself turning to food for solace, a poor substitute for love, companionship, and financial security. Amy's stress trigger was loneliness, and her response was to eat.

A New Angle

Many therapists find it useful for their patients to create a "bad habit genogram"—a kind of family tree of bad habits. In that way, a person can trace how a certain behavior, or pattern of behavior, develops through the generations and how such patterns now affect him or her. Certain habits, such as those that involve chemicals like alcohol and nicotine, may have a direct genetic link, while other children pick up bad habits by observing them in their parents or other relatives.

After she'd examined and understood her bad habit's roots, Amy realized that in meeting the challenge of breaking her bad habit, she also laid the foundation for a great deal of personal growth, and a new, deeper relationship with her mother.

Best of all, she could let herself off the hook: Amy didn't have a problem with food because she was worthless or weak. She had a problem with food because she learned, by example and by the power of oral history, that food *should* make her feel better.

What about you? Is it possible you learned your behavior from someone else close to you? Maybe you saw that one of your parents used to have a cocktail before dinner as a way to de-stress and disconnect from the hubbub of family life. Now, when you're supposed to be mingling at a party, you clutch a martini (or two) as if it were armor.

But the connection doesn't have to be so direct. Remember, the basic motivation for all bad habits is the same: Avoiding the stress of loneliness, anger, discomfort, and fear. Maybe one of your parents avoided stress by telling all of those "little white lies," for example, so you now pride yourself on your honesty and candor. Good for you! But boy do you procrastinate, or fly off the handle, or arrange your closet with a military orderliness when faced with one of your stress triggers. What you learned growing up was the art of avoiding a feeling or situation; you just chose a different mode of expression than your parents did.

Reruns with a New Cast

You know the old saying "Those who don't know history are doomed to repeat it"? When it comes to breaking bad habits, there's another step involved. Not only is it important to understand the roots of your bad habit, it helps to take the time to "recast" the images from your past that keep you from moving forward.

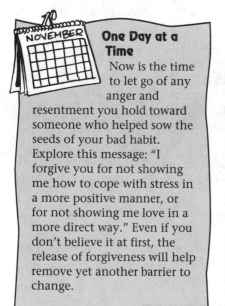

One Day at a Time

Now is the time to let go of any anger and resentment you hold toward someone who helped sow the seeds of your bad habit. Explore this message: "I forgive you for not showing me how to cope with stress in a more positive manner, or for not showing me love in a more direct way." Even if you don't believe it at first, the release of forgiveness will help remove yet another barrier to change.

In Chapter 4, "Okay, So How Do You Stop?" we asked you to start recording over any negative messages your mind keeps presenting as indisputable truths. You know, the ones that say, "I'm a failure" or "I'm weak." Here, we're asking you to reconsider where those messages come from and what they mean. When Amy plays back her mental videotape of coming home from school, for example, she should focus on the loving note her mother left for her rather than on the fudge brownie with ice cream. Just a small camera adjustment, and the picture changes. By making this minor realignment, Amy can—pardon the completely inappropriate cliché—have her cake and eat it, too!

Let's face it, though. What happened in the past to establish a current pattern of behavior is just that—the past. We're adults now and responsible for making our own choices. No matter how ingrained your habit has become, you still *choose* to perform it. The good news, then, is that once you truly discern the pattern, you can choose to *break* that pattern in the future.

Be Your Own Bad Habit Detective

You probably don't think much about what gets you through your day, but instead pass through it quite conscious of some things and only vaguely aware of others. More than likely, you're least aware of the very activity you most want to change: Your bad habit. You check your e-mail 18 times a day without making a mindful decision to do so. The lie about how much TV you watch (and which programs, too!) slips out before you have time to consider it. It's only at the end of the day that you realize your jaw is in a permanent clench and that instead of a daily eight glasses of water you've had a six-pack of assorted caffeinated beverages.

Clearly, you won't be able to break your bad habit until you recognize—before the fact—when you're about to perform it. Now, think about the very last time you indulged in your bad habit, and then fill in the blanks in the following exercise:

I...

➤ Bit my nails

➤ Max'ed out my credit card

➤ Ate the whole thing

Fill in Your Bad Habit: _____

When...

➤ The company president made my assistant my boss.

➤ The next-door neighbor I can't stand won the lottery and decided not to move.

➤ It rained all through my first vacation in two years—to Paris, no less!

Fill in Your Trigger: _____

Because...

➤ If I didn't bite my nails, I might consider strangling the company president and that's definitely not a good idea.

➤ If I didn't shop, the festering ulcer that living next to this neighbor has given me might perforate.

➤ If I didn't eat, what else could there possibly be to do in Paris in the rain? Louvre, schmouvre.

Fill in Your (Irrational) Reason: _____

The examples above are outrageous ones—most of them would drive anyone to carry out a negative behavior of some kind (ever hear of going postal?!). The kind of things that trigger most run-of-the-mill bad habits, on the other hand, are usually pretty minor: You're ten minutes late for work, your significant other forgets to kiss you good-bye in the morning, the bathroom scale shows you've gained a pound, you stub your toe in your new sandals. Things you probably wouldn't think twice about under most circumstances.

The next exercise, however, forces you to think about your behavior, hour to hour, day by day. You'll track what you think about, who you're with, and what motivates you to bum that cigarette, let three weeks of unfolded laundry pile up on your bed, head to Vegas to play the slots. Answer the following questions each time you perform your bad habit of choice:

1. *Who's around or who do you think about just before you do the bad habit deed?* Logical choices include:

   ➤ Your employer or coworker

   ➤ A family member (Pick someone, anyone! And don't leave out Fido, the family pet.)

   ➤ Nobody

2. *What are you doing just before you get your bad habit urge?* The range here is enormous:

   ➤ Lying in bed contemplating the day ahead.

   ➤ Staring at a bill marked past due in bright red.

   ➤ "Conversing" happily as always (not!)—with your ex.

3. *When do you indulge?* Sooner or later:

   ➤ Exactly three seconds after you notice the run in your stocking (or spaghetti sauce on your tie) as you sit in the reception area waiting to interview for a job. (Your neck cracks loudly to relieve the tension and the receptionist raises an eyebrow and congratulates you.)

   ➤ Three hours after your 6-year-old's second tantrum of the day. (You use butter instead of applesauce to enrich that cake batter.)

   ➤ A week after a blind date stands you up. (Gym clothes remain in the tote bag unused, again.)

4. *How did you feel as you did the dirty deed?* This is the biggie. Discovering what feelings stress triggers in you, and what you hope your bad habit will help you avoid or alleviate is essential. Could your bad habit be triggered by:

   ➤ Anxiety (which can feel like ants crawling on your skin or a vise cinching in your chest and abdomen).

   ➤ Depression (which presents itself not only in tearfulness, but also in *anhedonia*, or the inability to derive pleasure out of any activity).

   ➤ Boredom (which in its most entrenched state can *seem* like relaxation—i.e., the feeling you get when you're watching a fifth straight hour of television on Saturday night—but actually triggers as much stress as a Monday morning traffic jam). Being bored means you're frustrated and feel stuck, which are both stressful emotions.

By answering these questions for several days running, each and every time your habit takes hold of you, you'll be able to discern the pattern of behavior you've developed over the years in response to stress and other emotional triggers.

Your Daily Habit Log

To keep track of your habit in an orderly way, you might find it helpful to keep a "Daily Habit Log" where you write down your observations. It can take almost any form: You could use the same planner in which you keep your business appointments. On the other hand, if you're like most overworked information age citizens, you won't have room in there for the kind of details you'll want to notate. The best idea is to buy a regular old legal pad or copy book (remember the ones you had in school…?) and devote it to this, and only this, task of tracking down bad habits.

Strictly Speaking
Anhedonia is a psychological term meaning the inability to experience pleasure or a loss of interest in once pleasurable activities. Woody Allen originally wanted the movie *Annie Hall* to be titled *Anhedonia* because the main character (played by Allen) was such a malcontent!

Amy lent us this example from her Daily Habit Log. She set it up this way, using one page for each day.

Amy's Daily Habit Log

Monday	
Time	9 a.m.
Habit	Ate three donuts
Activity	Realized it was Saturday morning and I had no plans for the weekend
Feeling	Lonely, anxious, frustrated, sad
Time	2 p.m.
Habit	Pushed away salad at lunch; didn't eat at all
Activity	Meeting thin, married girlfriend
Feeling	Out of control, jealous, angry
Time	10 p.m.
Habit	Ate ½ pint of Häagen-Dazs Rocky Road
Activity	Watching *Baby Boom* for the gazillionth time
Feeling	Nothing at all

We hope you get the idea. You can add or remove any category that doesn't figure into your pattern—or change the log as you go along. If you notice that a particular person, or type of person (your sibling, specifically, or a procrastinator in general), then you might want to create a category like "The Usual Suspects."

Or you could decide to keep the log more like a journal, eliminating the need to follow such a strict template. It's really up to you. To help get you started for at least the first two days, though, we offer you this template based on Amy's example.

Read It and Weep

All the facts right up front, spelled out in a straightforward, easy-to-understand way. That's the goal of every journalist tracking a big story and every detective on the trail of a hot lead, and the questions listed on page 54 are the ones they ask first.

Today, you can think of yourself as your very own journalist tracking down your big bad habit story or, if you'd rather, a Philip Marlowe for the millenium on the trail of bad behavior. Your assignment: To track down those people and situations that stimulate your behavior.

Now that you have a plan of attack with your Daily Habit Log, you'll soon identify your personal bad habit pattern. Once you do that, you can work on finding ways to:

➤ Avoid the triggers;

➤ Alleviate the triggers before they reach their absolute threshold; and

➤ Find better ways to cope.

Mirror, Mirror on the Wall

If you use your Daily Habit Log consistently for more than a few days, a pretty clear picture will begin to form—not only of your bad habit, but also of your lifestyle, your emotional life, and the people and situations that may be holding you back.

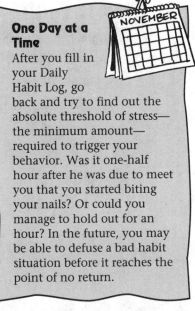

One Day at a Time
After you fill in your Daily Habit Log, go back and try to find out the absolute threshold of stress—the minimum amount—required to trigger your behavior. Was it one-half hour after he was due to meet you that you started biting your nails? Or could you manage to hold out for an hour? In the future, you may be able to defuse a bad habit situation before it reaches the point of no return.

Who's the person you see represented in those pages? The strong person you want to become? Or a person who's relinquished control over personal behavior to an outside force?

Don't you hate it when you're watching television and your partner has custody of the remote control? Even if you've agreed upon what to watch, you want to know you can change the channel, adjust the volume, or mute the commercials yourself.

That's what you want for yourself when it comes to the way you run your daily life. You want control over the choices you make. If you really *want* to bite your nails, you're at perfect liberty to do it. But if you want to have attractive hands and a calmer existence, you also can take control over the behavior that's preventing you from reaching those goals.

In Chapter 6, "Step 2: Evaluate Risks and Benefits," you'll proceed on to next step on your journey of change: Evaluating the risks and benefits of your habit and weighing them against your goals for the future and your sense of self-esteem.

Cold Turkey
Relax. No doubt you're excited about your journey of change, and that's terrific. But be careful not to let excitement become anxiety, or curiosity become obsession. Strong emotions of any kind (even good ones) are stressful, and thus potential triggers for unwanted behaviors, such as bad habits!

The Least You Need to Know

➤ You may have learned your bad habits as a way of coping in your childhood.

➤ Adjusting your view of the past, and forgiving others their past mistakes, will help you move forward.

➤ Keeping a Daily Habit Log helps you understand your bad habit and its triggers.

➤ You're now armed with the facts you need to retake control of your behavior.

Chapter 6

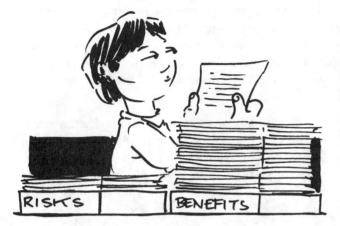

Step 2: Evaluate Risks and Benefits

The definition of insanity: Performing the same act, in the same way, over and over again—yet expecting to get a different result. Used by Alcoholic Anonymous, this definition perfectly describes how irrational a bad habit can be. Sogyal Rinpoche, an eminent Tibetan Buddhist master, approaches it from a different angle. Imagine you're walking down a street with a hole in the sidewalk and you step in it by mistake, wrenching your ankle. Not *your* fault. The next day, walking down the same street, you pretend you don't see the hole, but you end up stepping in it again. Still not *your* fault. (How dare that hole still be there!) The next day you walk down the street and step in the hole on purpose—it's a habit now!

And that's probably what's brought you to this book. You've realized one or both of the following things:

➤ Performing the same habit over and over again gets you the same negative result, over and over again. You can no longer say to yourself that *this time* the third cocktail won't cause you to lose control or that *this time* your tendency to prevaricate (i.e., deliberately misstate something) won't hurt someone else or undermine your own sense of integrity—because that's exactly what it did the last time you did it, and the time before that.

➤ Trying to break your bad habit by using the same method you've tried before (over and over again) with no success won't work this time either. You've quit smoking cold turkey six times before, but here you are again with a butt in your hand. Throwing "the last cigarette" down the garbage disposal and flicking the switch will not break your habit *this time* either, unless something else in your approach or your attitude is different.

And that's really why you're here—to discover a more positive and ultimately successful method of breaking a bad habit that's holding you back in some way.

So What's Stopping You?

Stress: It probably doesn't surprise you that making the final, ultimate, angst-ridden decision to break your bad habit causes you to feel anxious and under pressure.

But what's even more challenging, however, is living in the limbo of "maybe I'll quit, maybe I won't"; "I know I should, but a part of me still doesn't want to"; or "I know I should be able to, but I'm afraid I'll fail (again)." That state of indecision can be the most stressful of all. In fact, psychologists have studied this phenomenon in great depth, identifying three different types of conflicts that can arise from choice:

➤ **Approach-approach conflict:** When two equally desirable but mutually exclusive alternatives are presented.

Example: You love the way taking a drag on a cigarette feels *and* you love running five miles a day. You cannot do both any longer.

➤ **Avoidance-avoidance conflict:** When two equally aversive alternatives are presented, but both cannot be avoided.

Example: You bite your nails so far to the quick that they bleed sometimes. But the painful emotions that arise when you try to stop (the very emotions you bite your nails to escape!) are overwhelming.

➤ **Approach-avoidance conflict:** When a positive alternative is inseparably paired with an aversive one.

Example: You want to finish the project on time, even ahead of time, but to do it you have to stop procrastinating, concentrate, and block out all distractions—a tall order you find very difficult to accomplish.

When it comes to bad habits, most people grapple with the approach-avoidance conflict—they clearly see and desire the benefit (better health, prettier hands, increased productivity) but also realize how much they'll miss the habit, and thus resist making the change that makes the benefit possible (no more smoking, nail-biting, or procrastinating).

Experiencing those two emotions at the same time can be exhausting. In fact, that's probably how the process of rationalization became so popular. Instead of trying to hold onto two opposing thoughts or emotions—which creates a stressful consequence called *cognitive dissonance*—we alter one idea to make it less uncomfortable until we can bring our attitudes and behavior into alignment.

> **Strictly Speaking**
> Cognitive dissonance is a psychological term that describes the difficulty that occurs when your attitudes don't match your behavior. It's hard to accept both "I (an intelligent person) want to smoke" and "I know smoking is bad" as equally true. Instead, we fudge the truth and say, "Smoking isn't so bad," or "I'll quit tomorrow."

And how do we get rid of this dissonance created by the difference between what we think and what we do? By changing our behavior to fit our true understanding of the world and our place in it. If you believe you're a good, kind person, and yet know you have a tendency to lie, you ultimately have one of two choices. You can decide that you really are a *bad* person (and we bet you're not a bad person), or you can learn to stop lying and start telling the truth.

In Chapter 5, "Step 1: Identify the Behavior," you learned what kinds of situations or feelings trigger your bad habit(s). Right now, it's important that you take a good, hard look at just what you're getting out of that habit—for better, and for worse.

What's Really Good About Your Bad Habit?

There's no denying it. Your bad habit provides you with a certain amount of satisfaction and enjoyment. Generally speaking, performing your horrible habit helps you relieve anxiety by distracting you from difficult or uncomfortable feelings or activities. In addition, you probably derive some very specific on-the-spot benefits. Bad habits provide instant gratification.

61

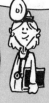

Strictly Speaking
Instant gratification is the thrill or burst of satisfaction you receive when you opt for your heart's—if not your mind's—desire. The bad news: The satisfaction is short-lived and the behavior attached to it often has long-term negative consequences.

These short-term benefits, rather than the overarching but intangible "relief from stress," may be what keeps you devoted to your bad habit, so it's important for you to identify what they are. Once you do, it will be easier to ensure that you are choosing your habits… and they're not choosing you.

In the Short Term

To get you started, let's take a look at the benefits one of our friends, Phoebe, a graphic artist, gets in the short term by procrastinating.

1. She doesn't have to concentrate or be creative.

2. She can think/do other things (like spending two hours on the computer figuring out some esoteric feature of PhotoShop or Quark instead of getting her work done).

3. She gets energy from being "naughty."

4. Feeling badly about herself and being self-critical is a "normal" state of mind for Phoebe.

5. She doesn't have to worry about whether anyone admires the illustrations she creates.

Whew! Just reading those "benefits" kind of takes the wind out of the procrastination sail, doesn't it? None of the so-called benefits support Phoebe's goals or nurture her sense of self.

Now, our trusted reader friend, it's your turn. Think about how it feels when you eat that high-fat, sugar-loaded snack; subscribe to your twentieth magazine; smoke that cigar; take your third bath or shower of the day; or push your partner's buttons during an argument. What pleasure do you *really* get from that behavior, right when it happens? Be honest.

Five short-term benefits I derive from my bad habit:

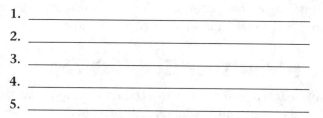

1. _____

2. _____

3. _____

4. _____

5. _____

What kinds of short-term benefits did you discover about your bad habit? If your habit of choice involved a substance, you probably focused on how good it tasted and how satisfied it made you feel on a physical level. A tendency like lying or losing your temper might provide you with a feeling of release (of tension or anxiety), or of control over an uncomfortable situation.

However, do you think that in the long run, these short-term benefits really hold up? Is it really worth it?

In the Long Run

Ahhhhhhhh. The long run. Here's where the "logic" of bad habits usually breaks down completely. Plainly speaking, most bad habits simply don't *have* any long-term benefits. Can you think of even one enduring advantage of overspending, for instance? Let's see. Maybe you'll have some nice clothes or furniture—unless they're repossessed for non-payment. Other than that, it looks pretty bleak. What about lying? You may have escaped some unpleasant situations, but the cost to your principles is very high. And smoking, well, if you count a mighty high risk of lung cancer as a long-term benefit, by all means, keep puffing away.

If you can think of any enduring benefits of your bad habit(s), write them down, too. The more you understand about what attracts you to your irresistible behavior, the better.

What's Really Baaaad About Your Bad Habit?

As their very name implies, bad habits have negative consequences. You know that already, or you wouldn't be reading this book. It will help you, though, to spell out exactly how your bad habit undermines your goals and sense of self—to see in black and white just how much your behavior is holding you back. Let's try it.

A New Angle

A 1997 survey conducted by CNN and *Men's Health* magazine revealed what doctors consider to be the most important good and bad habits when it comes to your physical well-being. The figure on the right represents the percentage of doctors who identified the habit as an important factor in determining health or disease.

Quitting cigarette smoking	98 percent
Avoiding illicit drugs	85 percent
Wearing a seat belt	81 percent
Avoiding high-fat food	55 percent
Eating a balanced diet	47 percent
Exercising at least 3 times/week	37 percent
Avoiding undue stress	26 percent

In the Short Term

Okay. This is the hard part. Instant gratification usually wins out in the short-term category—hands down. It's right there for you, you don't have to think about it, and it usually allows you to avoid experiencing a difficult emotion or performing a challenging activity. That's exactly how a bad habit seduces you into carrying out an action you know in your heart is ultimately damaging.

If you really think about it, though, and depending on your habit, you can probably come up with a few short-term negatives, too. Even though the instant benefits usually won out, for instance, Suzanne's friend James really hated having to trudge outside to have a smoke. And as much as Gary's former client Amy enjoyed eating a piece of cake, she didn't enjoy blowing her monthly budget on confections from her favorite gourmet bakery.

What about *your* bad habit? What do you dislike about it, just before or at the very moment you're performing it? Write it down. Remember it. It may come in handy later.

Five short-term disadvantages of my bad habit are:

1. _____
2. _____
3. _____
4. _____
5. _____

For the Long Run

If you've still got any doubts about breaking your bad habit, this next exercise should cast them aside for good. Here's where the romance and fantasy of a bad habit come smack up against harsh reality. Here's where you uncover some potentially unpleasant information about your life and the way you've structured it. Make no mistake: This ain't no disco, this ain't no party, this ain't no foolin' around.

Just to give you an idea of the kind of work involved, let's look at Phoebe's list of short-term procrastination "benefits" from a long-term perspective—to refresh your memory). The zoom lens on the videotape moves back to wide-angle, and here's what is revealed:

1. By avoiding her work, Phoebe is actually denying herself the opportunity to experience joy—the joy that comes from the act of creating. She's forgotten that, when it comes to art, it doesn't matter if she "accomplishes" or "completes" a project, the process itself is a joyful and fulfilling one.

2. There is also the issue of wasted time. Years can go by before Phoebe realizes that she already could have written and illustrated that children's book!

3. Whatever else Phoebe may do when she's supposed to be working, could it possibly be as meaningful? Maybe sometimes, but usually the time just gets frittered away on mindless activities like going out to the movies, which Phoebe can't even really enjoy because she's so worried about the work she's *not* doing!

4. Phoebe gets energy from being "naughty?" Not really. What she tells herself is that energy—the forbidden thrill procrastinators get from misbehaving—is really anxiety, anxiety that can lead to a few other bad habits, like overeating and over-spending.

5. Procrastination and self-criticism are often the masks of the perfectionist. If Phoebe feels she is never good enough, then procrastination becomes her excuse to avoid falling short of her own expectations for her talent. Chronic feelings of low self-esteem are at the root of many a bad habit.

6. Now, on top of her own feelings of self-criticism, Phoebe piles on everyone else's opinions, too.

There you have it: Fear of failure, fear of success, just plain fear. Except when it helps you move quickly from the path of an oncoming bus, fear is the most undermining emotion of all. Painful as it may be, uncovering these hidden bad habit motivations is a very positive step. It lays bare the emptiness of your bad habit and leaves little room for further rationalization. Let's look at some other damaging long-term effects of Phoebe's proclivity to procrastinate:

1. It undermines her professional credibility with her colleagues and clients.

2. It puts future projects on indefinite hold.

3. It keeps her from planning ahead, socially and professionally.

4. The fact that she's always working (because things tend to take longer than they should) annoys Phoebe's friends and family.

5. Procrastinating not only puts off Phoebe's enjoyment of her career, but it makes her unhappy and dissatisfied as a person.

There you have it. That's what Phoebe's bad habit *really* does for her. Nothing of value. Nothing of worth. Your turn. Take the proverbial bull by the horns and run with it. Explore your dark side, and then free yourself from it.

My Bad Habit Negatives

1. _____
2. _____
3. _____
4. _____
5. _____
6. _____
7. _____
9. _____
10. _____

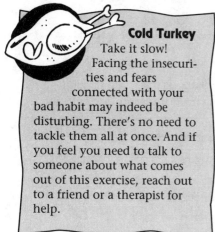

Cold Turkey
Take it slow! Facing the insecurities and fears connected with your bad habit may indeed be disturbing. There's no need to tackle them all at once. And if you feel you need to talk to someone about what comes out of this exercise, reach out to a friend or a therapist for help.

What did you come up with? Anything that made you think twice (or more than twice) about continuing your bad habit? After all, there's the possibility that after writing down the positive and negative effects, you could decide in favor of your habit. Maybe it really isn't so bad after all. As long as you're being really honest with yourself, you'll have made a valuable realization. If so, you can stop reading now, and simply accept your behavior as a healthy, or at least benign, part of your everyday life.

More than likely you've discovered your bad habit is an unnecessary burden. By freeing yourself from it, you'll be in a better position to maintain a healthy sense of self-esteem and attain your goals with more efficiency and less undermining anxiety. We say go for it—lose that nasty habit now!

What's the Worst That Could Happen?

The title of Chapter 8 (just in case you haven't already sneaked a peek) is "Step 4: Just Do It!" perhaps the three most frightening words to a potential bad habit breaker. Indeed, when you're this close to making a big, big change, all kinds of fears and anxieties probably sneak in. Most of them, fortunately, are completely irrational.

Let's see, death certainly isn't a usual side effect of breaking a bad habit. You will not die when you walk away from the next cigarette or turn off a cable TV shopping network or look your boss straight in the eye and admit making a mistake.

Failure isn't terminal either. So what if you fall off the wagon and start smoking or procrastinating again? As we'll discuss further in Chapter 9, "Get Back on That Horse," you'll probably learn a great deal from the experience of relapse, and the primary lesson will be that you can start over fresh, with new energy and commitment.

Another fear is of rocking the boat: What will your friends think if you choose club soda over beer at the next party? How will your sister feel if you can no longer be her binge-eating partner? What will you do with the extra time you have when you're no longer glued to the TV set? Does it mean you'll have to start exercising or volunteering at a soup kitchen?

How scary is it to finally take control of your own life and destiny? Pretty darn scary if you're like most mortals. But the benefits of taking charge of your life are innumerable. And you start to count them right now.

What's the Best That Could Happen?

Right now, congratulate yourself for making it through the difficult process of exposing your deepest insecurities and fears. We know it wasn't easy.

But now comes the good part: Imagining what life will be like without your bad habit. Remember that hole in the sidewalk we talked about at the beginning of this chapter? Well, think of that hole as a bad habit you are learning to sidestep. Soon, you'll be choosing an entirely different street to walk down. One full of exciting possibilities!

What you're really doing, of course, is turning your "My Bad Habit Negatives" into positives, which is the best way to incorporate them into your life. Instead of "Lying undermines relationships," consider "The truth creates trust and friendship." Instead of "Clenching my jaw is painful and uncomfortable," consider "I will relax my jaw and laugh more often."

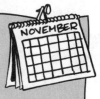

One Day at a Time
Breathe. Long slow breaths from the abdomen will relax you and help you focus. Close your eyes and breathe in deeply through your nostrils; feel your abdomen and then your lungs expand. Slowly exhale. Do this five times. Feel better? Deep breathing is rejuvenating and sends oxygen to the brain and internal organs—a natural high (and a very *good* habit to start)!

And, just in case you need even more incentive, you can take each benefit one or two steps further, creating a veritable ladder of success. For example:

"I will save money if I don't smoke."

"Having extra money means I can start paying off some debts."

"If I pay off my debts, I can start saving."

"If I start saving, I might be able to afford to take a real vacation next year."

If you can, make a ladder with a few of the benefits you consider the most crucial to your decision to break your bad habit. Once you finish, post the resulting ladder where you can see it. No doubt it'll continue to motivate you even during the tough times. In Chapter 7, "Step 3: Prepare for Change," we'll show you other ways to keep up your energy and commitment on your journey of change.

won't have to go to the bank so often

save money

be able to afford that special flavored coffee

feel more in control

If I stop smoking, I'll

start exercising

feel healthier

improve my skin tone

bring down my blood pressure

The Least You Need to Know

➤ You need to accept a new approach to change if you want to succeed at breaking your bad habit.

➤ Recognizing that there are good motives for your bad habits will help you find more genuinely healthful habits to cultivate.

➤ Carefully weighing the risks and benefits of your bad habit(s), over both the short- and the long-term, will help you recognize just how profoundly your bad habit(s) limit your life.

➤ It is important to let go of unrealistic fears and embrace the positive possibilities of breaking your bad habit(s).

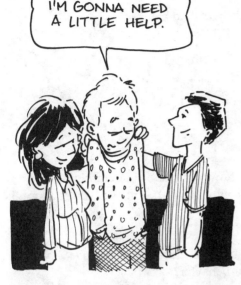

I'M GONNA NEED A LITTLE HELP.

Chapter 7

Step 3: Prepare for Change

In This Chapter

➤ Removing bad habit temptations

➤ Considering healthy good habit alternatives

➤ Asking and accepting help from your support system

How do you feel? If you've been doing the work we've asked of you so far, you've already made a quite a journey. Let's see just where you are in your own process of change:

Ready?

1. Do you recognize that a bad habit is undermining your goals or self-esteem?
   *Yes*_____   *No*_____

2. Have you identified the situations or people that trigger your negative behavior?
   *Yes*_____   *No*_____

3. Are you aware of the feelings you experience when you perform the habit, as well as the feelings the habit helps you avoid?
   *Yes*_____   *No*_____

Willing?

4. Do you fully understand the benefits and risks your bad habit offers?
   *Yes*_____ *No*_____

5. Have you decided that the risks outweigh the benefits?
   *Yes*_____ *No*_____

6. Are you willing to do what it takes to break your bad habit?
   *Yes*_____ *No*_____

Cold Turkey
The idea of having to "hit bottom" before you can make an important change in your life is a dangerous myth. Your life does not—we repeat: *does not*—have to be a complete disaster before you develop the strength and commitment to break your bad habit.

Able?

7. Do you know how to prepare your emotional and physical environment for the changes you're about to make?
   *Yes*_____ *No*_____

8. Are you able to concentrate on the positive aspects of changing your behavior?
   *Yes*_____ *No*_____

9. Do you have a support system of friends, family, colleagues, or others in place?
   *Yes*_____ *No*_____

How did you do? With any luck, you were able to answer "Yes" to most of these questions—at least until you reached the third category, which concerns the very important step of preparation. (If you answered "No" to more than one or two of the first six questions, you may want to revisit previous chapters or rethink your commitment to breaking your bad habit.)

Holding on to That Last Cigarette

The truth is, most people who try to break their bad habits but fail, do so because they don't take the time and effort to properly prepare themselves or their environment for the changes about to take place. They fail to consider the inroads, major and minor, that the habit has made into their daily lives and relationships.

Smoking offers some obvious examples: The extra packs of cigarettes hidden in various drawers; the ashtrays scattered throughout the house; the smell of tobacco lingering on your clothes; the craving triggered by your first cup of coffee. Then, of course, there are your still-smoking friends, coworkers, the person sitting at the next table in your favorite restaurant's smoking section (where you still ask to sit just to breathe it all in—idiot that you are!).

And, oh, the perpetual pleasure of that last cigarette! In 1923, Italo Svevo, an Italian author and a contemporary of Freud, wrote the first great novel about psychoanalysis called *The Confessions of Zeno*. (You remember Zeno's paradox: You divide something in half, and then that half is divided in half, and so on into infinity…making it impossible to achieve an end—like, say, breaking a bad habit.) The subject of the novel is this: The protagonist, Zeno, now an old man, is asked by his analyst to write down the reasons for his life-long love of smoking and why he feels he should stop. Here's what Zeno writes about the poignant pleasure of a last cigarette, and the next "last" cigarette, and the next "last": *The last has an aroma all its own, bestowed by a sense of victory over oneself and the sure hope of health and strength in the immediate future. The others are important too, as an assertion of one's own freedom, and when one lights them one still has a vision of that future of health and beauty, though it has moved a little further off.*

So, you may want to stop smoking, or stop whatever your bad habit of choice may be, but you aren't considering that breaking your bad habit means changing your life too! "Well, that's a bit much," you think. And so you linger in the doorway to change, spellbound by the last cigarette, clinging to the *hope* for change.

The urge to perform your habit does not go away through force of will. Your hands ache until you crack your knuckles. You can't concentrate until you've checked the stock market online—at four different Web sites. Your body feels like it will explode with tension until you drink that caffeinated beverage (caffeine to relax!!?!). Before you enter into the "action" phase of breaking your bad habit, you've got to identify those impulses and find a way to eliminate or modify them.

Let's examine the changes in your emotional, social, and practical everyday life that are likely to occur as you prepare to break your bad habit.

Accentuate the Positive, Eliminate the Negative

"I generally avoid temptation unless I can't resist it," said actress Mae West. And that about sums up temptation for most of us. If it's there before us, we have a hard time keeping ourselves in check, especially when it comes to an ingrained behavior pattern like a bad habit. It's right there, you know it so well, you remember (so well) how it feels to indulge, why not, *just this once,* I'll start again tomorrow…, I SWEAR.

Familiar feelings and words? We know, (we've been there!) and we don't blame you. It's perfectly normal—no matter how strong your commitment—to be drawn to the very behavior you've decided to eliminate. It's especially difficult when reminders and triggers, both physical and emotional, still surround you. The fewer temptations you have before you, the more successful you're likely to be.

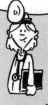

Strictly Speaking
Object permanence, knowing that an object continues to exist even when it's no longer perceived, is a stage of child development described by psychologist Jean Piaget. Take away and hide a two-year-old's pacifier, and the subsequent shrieking will be heard in China. She knows it still exists and she wants to suck on it NOW. Ring any bells?

It's important to note, however, that no matter how carefully you erase reminders and avoid triggers, you'll still have some bad moments. The fact is, as an adult, you've learned from experience that "out of sight, out of mind" is a cruel myth. Purging your office and home of all things caffeine doesn't erase the existence of the 16 coffee bars littering your neighborhood—or your knowledge of them—in fact, you learned the concept of *object permanence* when you were just a baby. Asking your family not to call and nag may help you avoid a few jaw-clenching incidents, but the memory of their concerns will still ring inside you, even if the telephone remains mute.

It makes sense to prepare your environment as best you can to accommodate and facilitate the changes you're about to make. Let's start with the physical.

Creating a Conducive Environment

Take a look around your home, office, and other areas where you spend time. Are there items that remind you of your habit or that make indulging in it easy? We'll be expanding on these suggestions—as well as providing you with substitutions and replacements—in the upcoming chapters dealing with specific bad habits. In the meantime, here are just a few suggestions to get you thinking about the direct impact changes in your physical surroundings can have on the success rate of breaking a bad habit:

For Overdrinkers

➤ If you drink at home, remove all alcohol from the premises.

➤ Make your home a relaxing, inviting place to be. If you're comfortable at home, you'll be less likely to want to drink there or to go out to a bar to drink.

➤ Buy new glasses just for the beverages you'll be substituting for alcohol. Throw away or pack away the glasses you usually use for alcoholic beverages. Get them out of sight.

For Caffeine Addicts

➤ Throw away your 12-cup coffee maker. If you intend only to cut down (and not cut out) your coffee drinking, replace it with a single-cup French press or single-serving "coffee bags" so you can brew just one cup a day.

➤ Have just one mug on your shelf or at your office.

➤ If you're able, move your desk at the office as far away from the coffee machine as possible. (If you can't move your desk, ask to have the machine moved.)

For Overeaters

➤ De-fat and de-sugar your kitchen. Search your refrigerator and cabinets for any foods you want to avoid, and then either store them in the freezer (under *plenty* of protective wrap) or toss them.

➤ Set the table with placemats and napkins at every meal. Sit down at the table to eat your food. Make mealtimes pleasant events.

➤ Remove the television from the kitchen and dining area. The combination of food and TV is the most undermining of all when it comes to controlling an eating problem.

For Nail-Biters

➤ Get a manicure so that your nails look as neat and attractive as possible.

➤ Wear gloves around the house for an entire day. If you're a woman, buy some colorful nail enamel, and leave the bottles on the bathroom counter to remind you of your goal.

➤ Place a picture of someone you admire shaking the hand of another person you admire on your refrigerator (say, Bill Gates and Steve Jobs, or Secretary of State Madeline Albright and former secretary Henry Kissinger): You can bet *their* nails are groomed with care. Not to mention Oprah's nails, Tom Brokaw's, or Barbra Steisand's…!

For Perpetual Slobs

➤ Spring for a maid or cleaning service—at least once—to get you started.

➤ Take a photograph of your home or office at its cleanest and neatest; tack it up on a wall that you pass often. Aspire to keep your environment that way.

➤ Throw or give away all unnecessary belongings. That means magazines more than a month old, clothes you haven't worn in two years, books you'll never open again, etc.

For Spendthrifts

➤ Cut up all but one of your credit cards (to use only in case of DIRE emergency). We know it hurts, but it's necessary.

➤ Dispose of all catalogs—for clothing, building supplies, hunting equipment, gourmet foods, pet accouterments, you name it.

➤ Consider blocking access to all home shopping networks on cable.

For Relationship Cheaters

➤ Put your little black book into the shredder.

➤ Erase all non-essential dates from your appointment book and replace them with solitary adventures or engagements with your mate.

➤ Dispense with any pager numbers, post office boxes, or online screen names you've used for your dalliances.

Get the idea? You want to feel as comfortable, as supported, and as free from temptation as possible during your journey of change. Clearly *every* habit doesn't require environmental changes to be broken. A congenital liar, for example, doesn't need any special equipment (except, maybe, a gullible idiot). Gamblers can generally avoid seeing a pair of dice, deck of cards, or slot machine simply by staying out of the casino. (Removing your bookie's number from speed-dial wouldn't hurt either!)

Take a look at *your* home or work environment. What can *you* change that will help you succeed in breaking your bad habit?

Five Things to Change at Home or in the Office

Things to Change at Home	Things to Change at the Office
1. _____	1. _____
2. _____	2. _____
3. _____	3. _____
4. _____	4. _____
5. _____	5. _____

Paving the Emotional Way

In the last chapter, "Step 2: Evaluate Risks and Benefits," we asked you to identify the positive and negative feelings your bad habit elicits. Since you're still reading this book, we'll assume the negative feelings outweighed the positive ones—convincing you that eliminating your bad habit may improve the quality of your life. And you've just listed things you want to eliminate from your physical environment to help you succeed in breaking that bad habit.

So enough with all the negatives and all the eliminations and all the precautions. Because the pull of your bad habit is likely to be very strong, it's important to give yourself more than a negative motivation to change. Think instead of how much you have to gain:

➤ **Self-respect.** You'll have even more reason to embrace your personal integrity and strength once you take control of your bad habit.

➤ **Sense of mastery and accomplishment.** Learning to live without your bad habit is just as difficult as learning any new skill—and just as rewarding. Think of how you felt the very first time you drove a car, conducted a conversation in a foreign language, or downloaded information from the Internet. Thrilled? Proud? You'll feel that way again when you master your bad habit.

A New Angle

In the mid 1990s, a group of researchers convened by the John D. and Catherine T. MacArthur Foundation of Chicago examined why people continue to engage in health-damaging behaviors. They found that people tend to act in proportion to their worries. In other words, long-term threats, however large, are less worrisome than immediate dangers, however small. One way to encourage yourself to change, the researchers found, is to concentrate on the *short-term positive benefits* of breaking your bad habit.

➤ **Material rewards.** Stop smoking a pack a day and see how much healthier you feel. Tame that gambling monkey on your back and maybe your bank account won't look so hollow. Stop lying and cheating and you might just get ahead in business. (Yes, ethical business people *do* make money!)

➤ **New horizons.** You won't be quite the same person once your habit is gone, which frees you up to explore new ways of being and feeling. You might even discover some talents and interests that were hidden in the shadow of your bad habit.

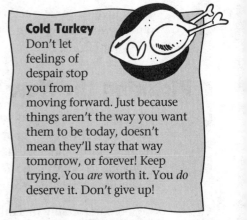

Cold Turkey
Don't let feelings of despair stop you from moving forward. Just because things aren't the way you want them to be today, doesn't mean they'll stay that way tomorrow, or forever! Keep trying. You *are* worth it. You *do* deserve it. Don't give up!

➤ **Fulfillment.** If your bad habit allowed you to attain all of your personal, professional, and social goals, you wouldn't be trying to break it now, would you? Imagine what you'll be able to accomplish without being held back by that pesky negative behavior, how rich and full your life could be.

Nurturing your inner life, your soul, is the best gift you can give yourself as you work to break your bad habit. Believe in yourself, listen to yourself, your deepest inner voice—the one your habit's been playing interference with. You may be surprised at what happens when you tune in to that frequency that is uniquely "you" and really start to pay attention.

With a Little Help from Your Friends

Ah ha! You knew something was nagging around that corner! What about your friends? Your colleagues? Your MOTHER???? How will *they* react? Can they really help or will they only hinder you? Should you tell them about your intentions to break your bad habit or not tell them?

Here's where it gets tricky and highly individual. Some people thrive in the spotlight. Others, though, only feel extra stress and pressure.

Three factors are involved in this matrix: The personality of the habit-breaker, the personality of the "supporters," and the relationship among them. If you're a naturally open person who finds it easy to share your struggles with others, have friends and acquaintances who appear to be the same, and you all get along well under stressful circumstances, then share away.

If you're more circumspect, however, you might want to confide only in a few close and understanding friends. It's especially helpful if you can find support among people with whom you spend a great of time, especially people who'll be there in the environment where you usually indulge your bad habit. If stressful situations at work trigger a tendency to avoid everything from meetings to picking up that phone that's been on hold for over a minute, for example, a workmate who can gently (and with your permission) help you stay on track can be a lifesaver. Do you have a sense of humor that allows you to take a little ribbing from your friends during the struggle? Or are you likely to become defensive? Being able to laugh at yourself—a little—and at your situation with others will certainly make the process of breaking your bad habit easier to bear.

As you prepare to take action against your bad habit, take time to think about who in your life will offer genuine support, and who might—even without meaning to—undermine your efforts.

Picturing the New You

Perhaps the very best way to prepare yourself for the changes to come is to imagine exactly how it will be—or at least how you'd like it to be—when your habit no longer interferes with your goals and sense of self. Remember the meditation exercise you tried in Chapter 2, "Why You Do the Things You Do"? Let's try it again—this time with a little visualization added in. You are the director: Lights, Camera, Action!

➤ Sit comfortably in a quiet room. Close your eyes. Take even, deep breaths. Let all the tension and stress flow from your body.

➤ When you've reached a calm state, begin to form a mental image of yourself as the strong, focused individual that you suspect you are inside. See yourself without your bad habit, in control and able to make sensible choices.

➤ Take another deep breath. Imagine yourself, strong and focused, in a situation that would typically tempt you to indulge in your habit. See yourself, clearly and precisely, choose another, healthier alternative.

➤ Finally, picture the result of your commitment, of how life will be without your habit dragging you down or holding you back. And don't be afraid to dream big. The sky's the limit.

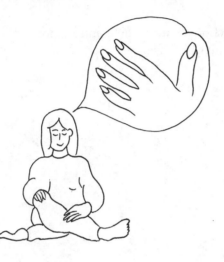

My nails are strong and beautiful.

Free, Free at Last!

You're approaching the moment when the idea of life *without* your bad habit becomes more compelling to you than life *with* it. That last cigarette isn't so poignant anymore. It's just dull and boring, yesterday's news. You're ready to put your own personal Sodom and Gomorrah behind you. (Try not to peek!) You've been there. You've done that. It's time for something new. Let loose your bad habit chains, and, (Now, where have you heard this before?) JUST DO IT!

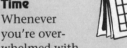

One Day at a Time
Whenever you're overwhelmed with memories of past failures or present insecurities, think of yourself as a programmable computer: Reprogram your hard drive with positive, life-promoting, joy-dispensing data and you'll automatically erase the undermining self-talk cluttering up your memory. Then you'll be able to perform the work necessary to break your bad habit much more effectively.

The Least You Need to Know

➤ Trying to skip a step in the process of change is liable to backfire.

➤ Improving your physical environment will help you adjust to the changes that will occur in your life, and help bolster your self-esteem.

➤ Focusing on the positive benefits you'll receive when you break your bad habit will help you succeed.

➤ Your friends may need direction about the help and support you desire from them as you journey down the path of change.

Chapter 8

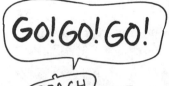

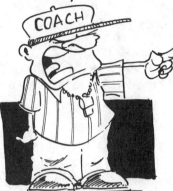

Step 4: Just Do It!

You've poked and prodded and explored your innermost feelings and motivations. You've identified your triggers and outlined your goals.

But the real hard work is yet to come. As writer G. K. Chesterton once so aptly put it, "There is a road from the eye to the heart that does not go through the intellect," and a bad habit knows that road very well. You can think, and think some more, about the ins and outs and ups and downs of your behavior, but you'll continue to perform the habit until you take very practical and deliberate steps to stop.

And now just might be the time to pull up your socks, bite the bullet, and get on with it. The very first thing you have to do is decide exactly when the action phase of your plan will begin.

And You're Off!

New Year's. Your birthday. The Summer Solstice. As soon as your three-year-old child enrolls in college. Tomorrow?

Just when *is* the very best time for you to break your bad habit? Sooner or later? Now or never? There's no easy answer. There's a fine line between choosing a comfortable time to break your bad habit and procrastinating endlessly.

Generally speaking, you'll have the best chance for success if you choose a date within a month after you've completed the prep work and made your final decision to break your bad habit. The longer you wait, the less successful your attempt is likely to be.

But the truth is, one day is pretty much as a good as any other when it comes to breaking a bad habit. Many people find that taking action on a Monday not only starts their week out with an energizing bang, but the busy days that follow help distract them from temptation. Others might choose a Saturday, when stress levels tend to be lower and more time is available for self-reflection and self-motivation.

Cold Turkey
Protect against procrastination! There will never be a "perfect" moment to make a dramatic change in your behavior. Life is complicated and it's bound to stay that way. Set a start date and stick to it. No excuses!

Only *you* know when you'll be ready to take action, and under what conditions you're most likely to flourish. You might find it terribly difficult to curb cravings for food or alcohol during the holiday season—most people do. On the other hand, if it's only August 1st, then start right in!

Take out your calendar, choose a date, draw a great big circle around it, and stick to it.

Baby Steps, Always Baby Steps

Does the circle you just made in your calendar mean you'll go to bed with a full-fledged habit and miraculously wake up without one?

Highly unlikely. Only if you've just acquired a very mild bad habit will it be possible for you to stop performing it all at once and once and for all. Fortunately, for the most part, taking such an all-or-nothing stance is unnecessary. Unless you have a serious and life-threatening addiction to alcohol or drugs, you may benefit from taking a more tapered approach than going "cold turkey."

Depending on how ingrained and demanding your bad habit is, you'll want to take a gradual approach to change. If you're drinking 18 cups of coffee today, it may be quite difficult—physically and emotionally—for you to drink absolutely no coffee on your start date.

Instead, create a more realistic and gradual plan of action. If your goal is to eliminate caffeine from your diet altogether, you can cut back from 18 cups to 14 cups the first day, and then one less cup per day until you no longer crave caffeine and you've successfully introduced healthier substitutes. (We discuss more about caffeine and its potential physical side effects in Chapter 13.)

Using a progressive approach doesn't mean you're any less committed to making a change than someone who goes cold turkey. Instead, it allows you to use time to your advantage. Remember, you didn't develop this habit overnight, so why expect to break it in such an unreasonable time period?

Taking baby steps helps you get through each difficult day in a sane and measured way. If you say to yourself, "I just won't drink a cup of coffee right now. Maybe I'll have a cup in an hour," you won't feel either out-of-control or deprived. When the next hour arrives, say the same thing again—"I'll just wait one more hour, and while I wait, I'll chew a piece of gum or take a walk." Before you know it, the day is over and you've made it without drinking any more coffee. But you'll have a whopping headache…. By setting small, reasonable goals, you'll increase your chances for success in both the short term and the long term.

The first hours, days, even weeks of breaking your bad habit are going to be tough. The short-term benefits (e.g., the relief of anxiety, the fleeting physical pleasure, the distraction from more serious issues) may *appear* to far outweigh the negatives (e.g., someday I might have a balance in my savings account or have an anger-free exchange with another driver on the freeway) at any given moment.

But "appear" is the operative word. And the long-term benefits of breaking your bad habit (potentially adding years to your life when you quit smoking and making them far more interesting by getting out of the house instead of watching TV all your life) are definitely worth more than the short-term benefits of your bad habit when you stack them up against each other. Remember creating your Ladder of Success in Chapter 6, "Step 2: Evaluate Risks and Benefits"? Go back and take another look at the goals you'll achieve if you actually succeed in breaking your bad habit. Live by it; that's right: LIVE BY IT! Make it real, one day at a time.

Getting Through It While You Do It

One day at a time? Eventually? This is a process? What about RIGHT NOW, when the urge to indulge in your bad habit overwhelms you? When you need to do SOMETHING or else you'll… Fortunately, there are plenty of practical, on-the-spot techniques available to help you through these bad moments.

The most important tool to help you stay on track while you break your bad habit is one we offered you back in Chapter 5—your Daily Habit Log. Remember?

Now, retitle your notebook: "My Daily Progress Log." This time, instead of writing down when you *perform* the habit, you'll be writing down when and how you *resist* the habit.

Here's how a Daily Progress Log might look for a coffee drinker on his way to a caffeine-free life.

My Daily Progress Log
Monday

Time: 8:30 am
Urge: To have a second cup of coffee
Trigger: Reading newspaper on-line
Feeling: Bored, dreading work
Strategy: Turned off computer,
              played with the cat

Time: 2 pm
Urge: To get a cappucino
Trigger: Impromptu staff meeting
Feeling: Tense, nervous
Strategy: Drank large glass of
              spring water

Time: 8 pm
Urge: Order an espresso
Activity: Out with Tom at
              favorite restaurant
Feeling: Like I deserved a reward
Strategy: Split a dessert and
              took a long walk
              through the park

One Day at a Time

It's easy to feel deprived and frustrated when you first cut yourself off from a familiar and comforting behavior. Keep in mind that having control over your bad habit gives you *more*, not fewer, choices. You're choosing to improve your life by breaking your bad habit; you're opening yourself to new opportunities.

The above example is just to get you started: Feel free to choose any format that works best for you. Many people find that keeping a full-fledged journal is more therapeutic than a simple log because it allows for more introspection and detail. No matter what format you choose, the important thing is to maintain it on a regular basis, especially at the start. Only if you're aware of when the urges to indulge occur, what triggers them, and what methods you use to avert them, will you be able to break free of your bad habit once and for all.

Finding a New Release

Most bad habits take energy to perform, energy you'll want to redirect into other, healthier behaviors. After all, your bad habit usually helps you to relieve feelings of anxiety or stress and these feelings trigger very physical responses within the body: your blood pressure and heart rate may rise, you may perspire more than usual, your gastrointestinal tract may do backflips. To some extent, your habit helps prevent or alleviate those symptoms, at least in the short term.

Finding healthy substitutes is a technique used in *behavioral therapy*, a particularly effective approach therapists use when helping people break their bad habits. Let's look at a few you might try.

One Day at a Time
Banish forever the idea of "willpower" as a tool required to break a bad habit or the armor you need to protect yourself against foreign enemies (i.e., temptation). Focus instead on taking control of the choices you make.

➤ **Healthy food.** Chewing on raw vegetables and fruit takes a lot of energy, keeps your mouth occupied (for those of you with a nail-biting, drinking, smoking, or eating problem, this is important!), and demands at least a little concentration and focus. Carry a baggie filled with your favorite low-fat, high-fiber foods and chew away whenever you get the urge to indulge in negative behavior. Set regular times for meals and allow yourself enough time to enjoy eating them. Add variety to your diet: If you eat only red meat, try adding poultry or fish for new lower-fat sources of protein.

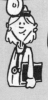

Strictly Speaking
Behavioral therapy is a type of psychological counseling that focuses on changing one's behavior in order to solve problems and improve the quality of life.

➤ **Paper clips and other toys.** Twisting a paper clip or fingering a coin can help distract you and occupy your hands. Make sure, though, that your fidgeting activity doesn't disturb others or you'll have a new bad habit to break!?!

➤ **New routines.** At least at the start, change the way you do things—even if it makes you feel uncomfortable. Altering your normal patterns can help eliminate your bad habit triggers. Here are a few suggestions:

Old Pattern	New Routine
Overeating at a restaurant	Eat a big salad beforehand
Smoking at a bar after work	Tea at a smoke-free cafe
Temper tantrums in the car	Listening to a book on tape
Failing to get to the gym	Walking briskly to and from work
Shopping after hard week	Planning a relaxing Saturday picnic

➤ **New endeavors.** Exploring a new activity or hobby—from knitting to rock climbing—can help direct your mind and body toward interesting new challenges. You won't have time for your bad habit if you're too busy learning, growing, and enjoying life.

➤ **Exercise.** A brisk walk not only takes your mind off your bad habit, it also may help release certain brain chemicals known to reduce symptoms of stress and anxiety. Get moving. Thirty minutes of moderate exercise every day can have a positive effect on your health (and on your outlook, too!). And remember—no pain, no gain is a myth; do what you can and stop when it starts to hurt. Build slowly.

➤ **A good night's sleep.** Scientists suspect chronic sleep deprivation can affect your immune system, hormone production, and short-term memory. Even one night of bad sleep can alter your emotional state, making you depressed, anxious, or irritable—which isn't a good state to be in when you're trying to break a bad habit. Set a regular schedule for sleep, going to bed about the same time every night. Stay away from caffeinated beverages after lunchtime. Only use the bed for sleeping—not working or watching TV. Take a warm bath before bedtime. Keep a bedtime journal; writing your fears and hopes in the journal may calm you so you don't stay up all night worrying about them!

Say a Little Prayer

Spirituality comes in all shapes and sizes, and means different things to all who embrace the term. What we mean by spirituality is a sense of faith—faith in the process of change, in the vitality of the human spirit, in yourself. Leave any cynical feelings behind and nurture your faith. Start here. Integrate these techniques into your efforts to break your bad habit.

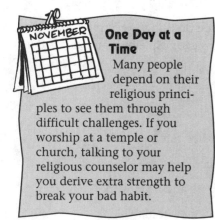

One Day at a Time
Many people depend on their religious principles to see them through difficult challenges. If you worship at a temple or church, talking to your religious counselor may help you derive extra strength to break your bad habit.

Meditation. In modern America, the ancient practice of meditation has emerged as a means of stress management because it allows people to let go of anxiety and fear while falling into a state of deep relaxation, peace, and tranquillity.

Remember the simple meditation exercise in Chapter 2, "Why You Do the Things You Do"? Didn't it feel great? Consider taking a meditation or yoga breathing class to help you disengage from the stress involved in breaking your bad habit.

Guided Imagery. Combining meditation and self-hypnosis, guided imagery relies heavily on the power of suggestion. In Chapter 7, "Step 3: "Prepare for Change," we asked you to perform *another* exercise (aren't we awful?!) where you first relaxed and obtained focus, and then imagined what your life would be like without your bad habit. That was guided imagery.

Another option is to imagine your habit as a dark cloud you can push away. Whenever you feel the urge to indulge in your bad habit, close your eyes, take several deep breaths, and picture yourself blowing that cloud—and that bad habit urge—away.

Hypnosis. Hypnosis is, more or less, a type of guided meditation. In a deep state of relaxation, your mind will hold onto subconscious suggestions such as "you no longer want to eat chocolate" or "smoking will make you sick" long after you come out of your "trance."

Tapes that use hypnotic techniques can be helpful in breaking bad habits, such as smoking, drinking, nail-biting, and compulsive gambling. Listen to a tape first during a meditation session and then while you sleep. Or make your own tape!

A New Angle

Many scientists believe hypnosis works by activating nerve pathways in the brain that cause the release of natural morphine-like substances called enkephalins and endorphins that modify behavior and help alleviate pain.

Rewards, Not Punishments

Remember how good it felt when your teacher put a gold star on a test you took or drawing you created? Or when your mom gave you an extra allowance for helping your dad clean out the garage all day Saturday? Those little rewards both encouraged you to keep up the effort and took the sting out of working so hard. They made you feel special.

Guess what? It's just as important for you to receive rewards for your hard work as an adult as it was when you were a child. In fact, since "go out and play" is a command rarely directed to anyone over the age of 16, adults are far more in need of "permission" to have fun than youngsters.

Now it's true that—eventually—you may feel stupendous when you choose a cup of soothing tea over a scotch or salad over beef stroganoff, or choose to paint the house or golf instead of run up your credit card. Right now, though, saying no to immediate gratification disappoints and angers you. You feel resentful and deprived, and for very good reason: You've lost your crutch, the one that held you up when anxiety, boredom, or just plain desire took hold.

It's essential to reward your effort—in big and little ways—throughout your journey. Link these rewards to meeting specific goals (a dinner out for a week of bad-habit–free living). Here're just few ideas to get your started:

Daily Rewards

➤ Positive self-talk ("Nice going" or "Good Job") for resisting an urge.

➤ Frequent relaxation breaks. (Two or three minutes during which you close your eyes, practice deep breathing, and, if you like, some guided imagery.)

➤ Taking a long walk in a different neighborhood.

➤ Slipping into a warm, scented bath at the end of the day.

Weekly or Monthly Rewards

➤ Tickets to a ball game.

➤ A weekly manicure. (Especially good for people trying to stop biting their nails, but actually a lovely treat for anyone!)

➤ Filling the house with flowers.

➤ Hiring a maid for a day and using the time to go to the movies, take a hike in a nearby park, or simply relax by reading a good book.

➤ Making a donation to charity or volunteering a few hours of your time.

Whenever you reward yourself, especially if you tie your treat to meeting a specific goal, record the reward in your Daily Progress Log. That way, you'll build a list of rewards that work to keep you bad-habit–free. And you'll have reminders of how much you've gained—not lost—since you've started to break your bad habit.

"I Don't Recognize You Without Your Bad Habit..."

You've come a long way and here you are, on your way to being bad-habit–free. Feels pretty terrific, doesn't it?

Maybe. Novelist and philosopher Anatole France once wrote. "All changes, even the most longed for, have their melancholy, for what we leave behind us is a part of ourselves. We must die to one life before we can enter into another."

This eloquent commentary on the effects of change may seem a bit dramatic to you, but you should take its meaning to heart. You are a different person than the one who bit her fingernails, or smoked, or fibbed, or ran up credit card bills at the hardware store. The difference may be dramatic, or it may be more subtle, but it's real.

A New Angle

As strange as it may seem, you may well experience sadness and even grief as you let go of your habit—and for three reasons. First, your habit was your "friend" for months or years and no doubt you'll miss it once it's gone. Second, you also may grieve for your old habit-loving self, the one you've been for so long. Finally, you may react with sadness when you come face to face with the feelings or situations you've tried to avoid by performing your now defunct bad habit.

The people you work with and the people you love may have a hard time adjusting to the "new" you. Even though they're cheering on your efforts to break your bad habit, they may also grieve for the person they're used to. You'll have to give others the space and time to accept the changes you're making. If you've decided to cut back on alcohol, stand by your resolution to drink only club soda at business luncheons. If you're trying to lose weight, don't let a friend talk you into a high-fat dessert "just this once." Saying no the first time may be hard, but others will come to respect your decision to break your bad habit. Who knows, they may admire your tenacity so much that you'll inspire them toward positive change as well!

Okay. We know what you're thinking. "What happens if I fail? What if I fall off the wagon? What if I just don't make it through the day without succumbing? What will people think? How will I be able to believe in myself?" Our answer to your concerns is: So what? Who cares? So you make a mistake. You're only human. It's not the falling down that matters—it's the *staying* down. Rocky Balboa never won a fight by giving up. Tenacity means persistent, stubborn, obstinate, tough. Put these words on index cards and post them on mirrors around the house. Pretty soon both you *and* those around you will start to define you in terms of your efforts to break your bad habit—not in terms of your old, bad-habit–loving self. Instead of "stuck" they'll call you "adventurous," instead of "hopeless" they'll say you're "brave." This new positive self-image will take on a tenacity of its own.

The Least You Need to Know

➤ Choosing an appropriate "start date" to begin breaking your bad habit will increase your chances for success.

➤ It's important to set small, attainable goals on your journey of change.

➤ Take advantage of the many techniques, including meditating, substituting healthy behaviors, and reaching out for support, to help you break your bad habit.

➤ Eating well, exercising regularly, and getting enough sleep are important aspects of creating a healthy life for yourself—with or without your bad habit.

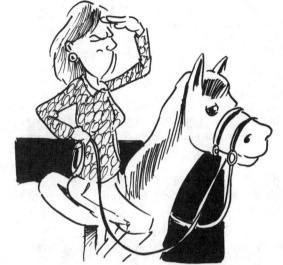

Chapter 9

Get Back on That Horse

In This Chapter

➤ Your risk for relapse

➤ Coping with the urge to be baaaad

➤ Making a new commitment to change

This chapter is about a topic that probably worries you a great deal: Relapse.

Fortunately, at the end of the day, a relapse isn't such a terribly big deal in most cases. Really! That's especially true if you've done all the up-front work necessary (understanding the roles habits play in your life, identifying your own bad habits and their triggers, etc.). You did the work, didn't you? And you're absolutely, positively sure that breaking your bad habit is what you really want to do. You are, aren't you?

If you answer yes to both questions, then don't despair. Here's the truth: Setbacks are a part of the process of change. They represent nothing more than a temporary blip on the bad-habit radar screen. Relapses may be disappointing and frustrating, but they're not a sign of failure or terminal weakness.

It's what you do next that's crucial. If you slipped and bummed one cigarette yesterday, does that give you "permission" to buy a pack and smoke it today (and be right back where you started from next week)? Or does it mean that you take a deep breath, look at all the progress you've made, and recommit immediately to having a habit-free future?

That's the question we'll help you answer in this chapter.

Like a Wave Crashing on the Shore

You're sitting at your desk at the office, facing an overflowing "in" box. The phone rings, and it's your significant other, nagging you about some argument you had this morning about the missing toothpaste cap.

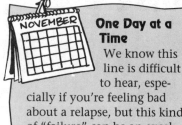

One Day at a Time
We know this line is difficult to hear, especially if you're feeling bad about a relapse, but this kind of "failure" can be an excellent opportunity for soul-searching and positive growth.

Before you know it, your hand moves to the computer keyboard. You don't mean to do it, you promised yourself you wouldn't, you'll only do it for a second, you've GOT TO DO IT RIGHT NOW… There it is: the Internet, ripe for surfing. How you've missed it. How you need it, just this once.

When next you look up, two hours have passed. An untouched pile of urgent interoffice memos are tilting precariously on top of the pile in your in-box, your message light is blinking wildly, and your boss is standing in your doorway, glaring. But you just found a cool Web site for the Hubble telescope!

Why did everything come crashing down when you were doing so well? Where did that urge come from, building in your body like a wave, and why did it overwhelm you at this particular moment in your day, your week, your life?

A New Angle

If you've suffered a relapse, you're far from alone. A 1995 study performed at Chicago's Loyola University Medical Center found that only 38 percent of people who make New Year's Resolutions stick to their plan a week later. After six months, the number dwindles to less than 15 percent. What does that say? Change is hard. (As if you didn't know!)

There are several potential answers to those questions, and none of them involves weakness on your part. The truth is, you're on an incredibly challenging journey and there are bound to be some rough waves to navigate as you make your way. Urges are indeed like waves crashing on the shore—just one big one can come up unexpectedly and ruin a perfectly peaceful picnic on the beach, or they can come at you one after another, after another, during a storm of anxiety and stress.

The challenge for you now is to learn from your relapse (You just knew that was coming didn't you?) and move forward. Let go of your anxiety, guilt, and despair by figuring out just what went wrong and why.

Relapse Traps: Which One Did You Fall Into?

Carefully review the Daily Progress Log we asked you to set up in Chapter 8, "Step 4: Just Do It!" You ARE still maintaining your log, aren't you? If you aren't, then you already know one reason why you've had a slip-up. Keeping track of your challenges, your triggers, and how you tackle them is an integral part of the process of change. Once you toss that aside, you're basically rowing upstream in a rudderless craft, without direction or power.

The following questions will help you track down the relapse culprit.

Has your life become more stressful?   *Yes*____   *No*____

Without question, additional stress caused by a change in jobs, a divorce, other relationship problems, or a death in the family, is the primary reason most people "fall off the wagon" of a habit-breaking commitment. When you think about your recent stress levels, keep in mind that stress takes many forms: Frustration, loneliness, boredom, low self-esteem are all common cohorts to the feelings of being overwhelmed stress usually causes.

Have you set unrealistic goals? *Yes*____   *No*____

Trying to do too much too soon is another common and deadly pitfall when it comes to breaking bad habits. Remember: Baby steps, always baby steps. If you can *never* play just one computer game, you should remove the temptation altogether by deleting the program from your computer. You're expecting too much from yourself if your bad habit is easily accessible, sending out its seductive siren call all day, every day.

Are you returning to the scene of the crime or consorting with the enemy?
*Yes*____   *No*____

"Come with us to the bar," say your well-meaning former drinking buddies. And you go, thinking that you'll have just a club soda instead of your usual scotch. Remember how important it is to avoid triggers of all kinds, including people (your nagging parent, your incompetent assistant), environments (like bars, smoke-filled restaurants), and situations (lonely Saturday nights, overscheduled work weeks) that push your "habit buttons."

Do you feel unworthy or guilty? *Yes*____   *No*____

In our opinion, the fear of success is as undermining to the action stage of breaking a bad habit as fear of failure is to getting started in the first place. Just when you start to feel

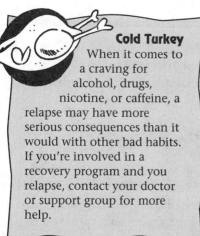

Cold Turkey

When it comes to a craving for alcohol, drugs, nicotine, or caffeine, a relapse may have more serious consequences than it would with other bad habits. If you're involved in a recovery program and you relapse, contact your doctor or support group for more help.

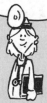

Strictly Speaking

A person who **internalizes** incorporates a new attitude because it largely agrees with his or her system of values: You don't lie because you feel in your soul that lying is wrong.

A person who **complies** changes behavior to conform with outside pressure from family, friends, or community: You stop lying—at least for a time, but don't really believe that lying is wrong.

stronger and more in control it hits you: "I don't deserve this. I'm not a strong person. I'm unworthy! I may be fooling other people who think it's so great that I don't smoke anymore, but I know that inside I'm still worthless. So I'm just going to smoke again…"

And there's the trap. These feelings of worthlessness trigger one of two things: a need for comfort or a need for punishment. Either way, your bad habit is waiting in the wings, itching to take precedence in your life again. Before you know it, you have found the "perfect" reason to reindulge.

Do you think you can "eat" just one?
Yes____   No____

Just one hour on the Internet, just one bite of cake, just one little white lie. We've all said it to ourselves, but we're rarely able to stick to that prescription. Face it: If it was a bad habit before, it's highly unlikely that you'll be able to control the behavior now, especially if you're relatively new to your habit-free life.

Did you think you were "over it"?   Yes____   No____

Ah, the old experiment trap: "Let me just see if I'm over this bad habit. I'll try just a little to check." Let me see if I'm over it yet. It starts out like an experiment, like the coffee drinker who's sure he doesn't need that cup of Joe anymore and wants to "prove" it to himself.

Did you break your bad habit for the right reasons?
Yes____   No____

Your doctor wants you to stop smoking, your significant other wants you to lay off the computer, your kids make fun of your eating habits, your best friend is tired of your lies and evasions… and so, you break your bad habit to please them. If you break your bad habit simply to please or assuage someone else (called *compliance*), and not because you believe it truly is best for you (called *internalization*), you're simply inviting failure.

Do you remember to reward yourself?   Yes____   No____

Feeling deprived of comfort and love—and then making up for that loss by indulging in your bad habit—is a very common reason for relapse. Review the section in Chapter 8, "Step 4: Just Do It!" about rewards, and make sure you find ways to treat yourself well throughout your journey of change.

Did answering these questions help you figure out what caused your slip? We hope so, because that way you may be able to protect yourself from a future relapse. For now, however, stop analyzing the situation and move forward.

Calling Back the Troops

Knowledge is power, right? We've said that before, and we warned you we'd say it again. Now you know. Your bad habit may be on its way out the door, but it isn't gone for good, at least not yet. You'll still experience urges, but at least you know how you can avoid them a bit better.

➤ **Review and reevaluate your triggers.** Stay faithful to the process of change by maintaining your Daily Progress Log. Explore what triggers your urges and how you can better avoid those people, environments, and situations.

➤ **Reaffirm your commitment.** Make sure you really want to break your bad habit, and that you want to do it for the right reasons. If you're not ready to address this problem now, wait until your circumstances and commitment is solid.

➤ **Relearn strategies to resist urges.** Practice makes perfect, especially when it comes to making behavior changes permanent.

Purge the Urge

When your bad habit urges surge, purge! Here's how:

Admit the Urge. First of all, accept that you have the urge, no matter when it occurs. Don't lose patience with yourself, whether the urge happens just two hours after you first break your bad habit, or weeks after you thought you'd licked your bad habit for good.

Detach from the urge. Look at your urge as something separate from you, something that you can study and dissect, or simply push away. You're the boss.

Personify the urge. You might find it easier to gain control over your urge if you classify it—the Inner Brat, My Old Self, the Thing—and then call it by its name whenever it threatens to upset your equilibrium. Again, the idea is for you take command of the situation.

Talk back to the urge. If the urge to indulge starts to sweep over you (and it will, especially at the beginning), tell it (forcefully) to go away. Say it out loud it you need to.

Remind yourself that the urge will pass. Every day you successfully suppress hundreds of major and minor urges—to scream at your boss, to filch an extra newspaper from the kiosk, to eat the entire box of donuts before you get home from the store. This urge is no different: The consequences are simply not worth the momentary pleasure and release of indulgence.

Distract yourself from the urge. At the start, this approach may help you the most. Instead of giving in, substitute another behavior to take your mind off the urge or craving. Here are just a few healthful suggestions:

➤ Close your eyes, take a deep breath, and relax. This action will help release your anxiety.

➤ Take a break from the trigger. So frustrated with your work that you reach for a cup of coffee? Leave your desk for five minutes, or concentrate on another task until your frustration, and the urge, passes. Or have a cup of tea—most teas contain less caffeine than coffee does.

Imagine a negative outcome—and the more negative and graphic, the better. If drinking one too many glasses of wine at a business lunch is your problem, imagine losing the whole deal—or even your job—because you lost focus. If you're trying to avoid losing financial control, imagine bouncing your mortgage payment or having to ask your parents for a loan.

Staying the Course

The message of this chapter is simple: Relapse is a natural part of the process of change. It doesn't mean you've failed or that you're weak. Each time you relapse, you'll learn something new about yourself, your strengths, and the stresses and strains in your life that challenge you. You'll know better what works and what trips you up. It will get easier, and the urges will lessen—as long as you get back on that horse and keep riding toward a bad-habit–free future.

To help you see the big picture, we suggest you go to a stationery store and buy a box of gold star stickers. Put a star on every day—either in your Daily Progress Log or on a regular wall calendar—that you manage well, that you either succeed at resisting an urge or learn something important about your motivation and commitment. At the end of the week, month, and then year, you'll be able to review the remarkable progress you're making—a star-studded universe of inspiration.

The Least You Need to Know

➤ Relapse is a natural part of the process of change.

➤ Urges and cravings do not disappear right away...or ever.

➤ Tracking down the reasons for your relapse now will help you protect yourself against future relapses.

➤ Relapse does not mean failure, but simply another opportunity to learn and to grow.

Part 3
Resist Those Cravings

We want what we want when we want it, as the old expression goes. When it comes to your relationship to certain substances, however, indulging your desire can be undermining and often quite hazardous. In fact, there's a fine line between bad habit cravings, dependencies, and addictions when it comes to substances like alcohol, nicotine, caffeine, and even certain foods.

In this part of the book, we outline the effects these substances have on the body. We also help you weigh their risks and benefits. And if you decide that you've got a bad habit you want to break in this area, we'll show the best ways to gain control over alcohol, nicotine, caffeine, and food.

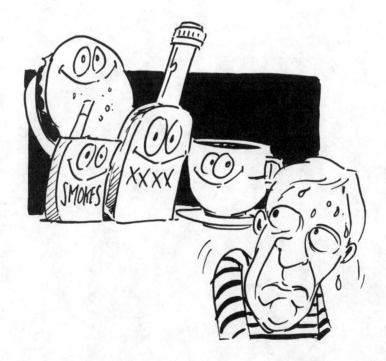

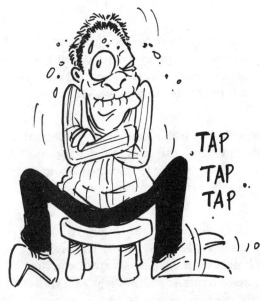

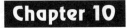

Identifying Your Cravings

TAP
TAP
TAP

In This Chapter

➤ What's so constant about cravings?

➤ How cravings target the mind *and* the body

➤ When willpower is not enough

Do you smoke cigarettes? Then we bet you'll tell us—as most smokers do—that few things are more satisfying than that first cigarette in the morning or the one right after dinner. How about the pleasure of a good bottle of wine with your meal followed by an Irish coffee or a fine port or cognac? Or a six-pack while watching a ball game? Or an ice cold soda at the beach? What about the rich aroma and focusing jolt you get from coffee before a breakfast meeting at work? And food: Well, from the guilty delight of donut-munching by the refrigerator light at 3 a.m. to a sumptuous seven-course feast, food is what sustains us and nourishes our bodies.

The Nature of a Craving

Desire. Need. Satisfaction. Pleasure. All natural, basic instincts and responses every human and most animals experience on a daily (maybe even hourly) basis. Craving is a good thing! Craving is healthy. When we eat or ingest any substance the primal goal (Yes, we do have primal goals...even in the twenty-first century!) is to stay alive. We crave nourishment, and nourishment gives us pleasure.

We have other instinctive cravings, too. Psychologically, we all require love, support, and comfort from the people around us so our hearts and minds can grow and develop in a healthy way. If you doubt that people really do need people, just look at the joy and reassurance a baby gets from its mother and father. The joy of human contact begins at birth and continues throughout our lives.

In today's fast-paced, stress-filled world, our primal cravings seem easily met. We don't have to hunt and gather food anymore (at least not in America, we don't); we just go to the supermarket, shell out some cash, and food is ours for the taking—convenient, pre-packaged, and ready for the microwave. Anything we want. As ads for the phone company tell us every day, love—communication with another human being—is just a call, a fax, or an e-mail away. And we don't need a wagon train to reach out and touch someone; we have trains, planes, and automobiles. It's all so easy—maybe too easy. Alcohol, nicotine, caffeine, and foods from all over the world—in or out of season—are at our fingertips all year long. Nothing is a luxury anymore. We live at a perpetual feast table, complete with advertisers to whet our appetites for each delight.

So when something isn't going right in our lives, when something happens that throws us off balance or makes us feel stressed out, a world full of plenty can turn into a world full of temptation. We look for the guaranteed, unconditional pleasure, the quick high substances like caffeine, nicotine, alcohol, and certain foods can offer us. After all, caffeine gives us the gift of concentration when we need it, without a lecture for being late or procrastinating. A glass of wine relaxes and comforts us, without asking us to reveal the source and cause of our distress the way our spouses most certainly would. The sugar-fat high of a pint of ice cream becomes a bottomless pit of love we eagerly dive right into. And that tenth cigarette of the day, well it's just what we *need* to get us through.

When You've Just Got to Have It

"An unfortunate thing about this world is that the good habits are much easier to give up than the bad ones." Writer W. Somerset Maugham knew what he was talking about. When it comes to substances such as alcohol, nicotine, caffeine, and food, for many biological and psychological reasons, bad habits are easy to develop and among the toughest to conquer. When you indulge, you feel good. That's because the chemicals that make up these substances trigger very real, physical, and—at least at first—pleasurable changes in the brain. So when you attempt to break a bad habit related to a substance, you're fighting a battle on two fronts—one in your mind and one in your body.

A New Angle

Although we tend to associate addiction with chemicals like nicotine and alcohol, scientists at Rockefeller University have isolated at least two chemicals in the brains of rats that convey very precise and compelling commands to the body about food. One chemical called galanin, underlies a yen for fat, while another called neuropeptide Y causes carbohydrate cravings. The more of each the body produces, the stronger the drive is to eat those particular food groups. However, they also noted that at least 25 other neuropeptides affect food intake, making appetite one of the most complex systems in the body.

Is It All in Your Head?

It's true: Some people can drink just a little bit, take or leave caffeine, and only eat when they're hungry. An extremely rare few can even smoke a few cigarettes and then leave the pack behind in a heartbeat. At the other end of the spectrum, we've all heard stories about, or known someone, who lived to be ninety and who smoked, drank, or ate, whatever she or he pleased, whenever she or he pleased.

But most of us just aren't quite so "blessed" in either direction. For millions of people, cravings for these benign substance turn into greedy bad habits, sometimes slowly over time, sometimes quite suddenly. The components of wine, beer, liquor, cigarettes, cigars, coffee, cola, and all foods can be broken down into powerful chemicals that produce profound effects on your body—effects that often make it difficult to resist the urge once you get into the habit of ingesting them. So, is it all in your head? Well, yes and no. The power of the feelings you begin to associate with what you eat, drink, or smoke combined with the chemical effects of these substances on your body, is what gets you into trouble. Let's take a closer look at the ways eating, drinking, or smoking can affect you on an emotional level:

➤ **Comfort and love:** Feeling lonely on a Saturday night? Have a big plate of pasta. Or a beer. Or a smoke. (But how long before comfort slides over into disgust?) Stressed out a work? Pour another cup of coffee; just the feeling of the cup in your hand makes you feel more secure (until the jitters set in, you can't seem to concentrate anymore, and that acid feeling settles over your stomach).

➤ **Reward:** Make that big deal at the brokerage? Get through a rough week with the kids? Then you've *earned* that second (or third) martini on Friday night. (But is the hangover the next day really the reward you deserve?)

➤ **Stimulation:** Feeling droopy in the evening? A caffeinated diet soda will perk you up. (But what about when it's 3 a.m. and you still can't get to sleep? Maybe scarfing down that last donut will help?) Bored and drained? Grabbing a beer and a smoke at the local bar might just get you going. (Until you realize your family hasn't seen you in a week!)

➤ **Relaxation:** You always feel tense and anxious at parties, but munching away at the hors d'oeuvres calms you right down (except that the weight you put on will only make you feel even more insecure at the next party). So does clutching that cigarette (even though your hostess makes you smoke it outside, defeating the purpose of being at the party in the first place).

➤ **Distraction:** Can't face what's really bothering you? Eat. Drink. Smoke. Crank up on caffeine. But is it really the easy way out, or a trap that leads to even deeper and more troublesome challenges down the line?

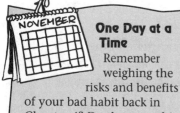

One Day at a Time
Remember weighing the risks and benefits of your bad habit back in Chapter 4? Do the same thing the next time want to indulge a craving: Balance the long-term negative emotional and physical risks against your bad habit's immediate benefits. Keep track of it all in your Daily Habit Log. You might just decide to resist!

Your first emotional challenge in attempting to break bad-habit cravings is to consciously understand the difference between satisfying a normal urge for nourishment and greedily indulging passionate, uncontrollable urges for excess. It's that ever-present tension between "want" and "need." It's knowing that having just one and the pursuit of the whole enchilada are two different things.

But there's another challenge here too: The challenge of taking responsibility for your pleasure away from the substances you imbibe and reinvesting it in yourself. It may seem difficult at first, but doing so will result in almost immediate physical and mental health benefits. In fact, as soon as you start really believing you can do it, and believing that you *are* worth it, the process of change will become easier to manage.

Or Is It a Chemical Thing?

Your body operates through a complex relationship of chemical processes that control everything from digestion to replacing body cells. So it seems reasonable that the substances you put into your body will affect the way it works—for better or for worse. Jack LaLanne, that fitness guy from the 1950s, compares good nutrition to putting premium fuel in an engine. But there's even more to it than that. Some of your body's chemical reactions take place in a part of the brain called the *limbic system*, the part involved in emotions, memories, and feelings of pleasure and satisfaction. Here's where the effect of cravings on the mind and the body blur into a Catch-22 that makes physical addictions so hard to break.

No matter what the substance, the basic pattern of a craving is the same: a recursive loop (kind of like a figure eight). A short time after you ingest a substance, you experience a period of satisfaction or pleasure. That's because the substances attach to certain receptors in the brain that trigger these good feelings.

> **Strictly Speaking**
> The **limbic system** is the part of the brain scientists believe lies at the heart of memory and emotion. It is made up of several different structures, connections, and neurotransmitters (brain chemicals) that work together. Dopamine is the brain chemical most linked to addictive cravings.

Unfortunately, this sense of gratification is usually short-lived and often followed by a dip in mood and then renewed cravings. In some cases, the loop recurs with specific timing that depends on how long the particular substance triggers changes in the brain. In smokers, for example, the nicotine loop can be as short as 20 minutes (which explains why it's so easy to smoke a pack of cigarettes, or more, a day—every 20 minutes your craving is triggered again).

Scientists have discovered that the same system involved in cravings is also responsible for providing a sense of pleasure whenever you find something rewarding, including having sex, eating chocolate, or completing a job well done.

It's no wonder we reach for cigarettes, alcohol, nicotine, caffeine, or food whenever we feel bad: They're designed to make us feel good in a hurry, and that's a tough proposition to turn down, especially when we're feeling emotionally vulnerable.

When Willpower Is Not Enough

There's a fine line between a bad habit—a repetitive behavior that has negative consequences—and an addiction, a bad habit that virtually takes over your life and which causes you physical and emotional trauma when you stop indulging in it.

There are several signs that addiction is beginning to take hold. If you start noticing that you *need* a drink after a stressful day, or that you're only able to soothe or satisfy yourself by overeating, your emotions are leading you down that slippery slope. If you notice that when you stop drinking coffee or alcohol you experience symptoms of withdrawal—irritability, shakiness, depression, nausea, for example—then your body has become physically addicted. It's no stretch to figure out that "just saying no" isn't going to sound very convincing to a body that's hooked on a chemical high. That's why it's so hard to break this particular brand of bad habit. That's why willpower just isn't enough.

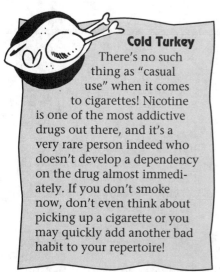

Cold Turkey

There's no such thing as "casual use" when it comes to cigarettes! Nicotine is one of the most addictive drugs out there, and it's a very rare person indeed who doesn't develop a dependency on the drug almost immediately. If you don't smoke now, don't even think about picking up a cigarette or you may quickly add another bad habit to your repertoire!

Evaluate your current use of substances to rule out the possibility that you've got more than a bad habit on your hands. Answer the following questions as honestly as you can:

1. Do you ingest more alcohol, cigarette smoke, caffeine, or food than you intend to on a regular basis?
   *Yes*____   *No*____

2. Have you tried to quit your negative behaviors related to a substance in the past but were overwhelmed by persistent desires or cravings?
   *Yes*____   *No*____

3. Do you give up other things in order to indulge your craving?
   *Yes*____   *No*____

4. Do you continue on a course of negative behavior, even though you know it's doing harm to you and/or your relationships?   *Yes*____   *No*____

5. Have you ever felt symptoms of withdrawal when you've tried to stop using the substance?   *Yes*____   *No*____

6. Have you ever experienced a black out after drinking?   *Yes*____   *No*____

7. Do you need more and more of the substance to achieve the same level of pleasure or satisfaction?   *Yes*____   *No*____

If you've answered yes to more than a few of these questions, your relationship to a substance such as alcohol, nicotine, caffeine, or food, may have become problematic. If that's the case, you should talk to your doctor or to another health professional as soon as possible. At the very least, you've got yourself a bad habit that's worth breaking.

Up on the High Wire

Balance. The acrobat walking the high wire across the chaos of Niagara Falls fills us with wonder, excitement, dread, fear, respect. That acrobat gets our adrenaline pumping. It's daring, it's wild, it's out there. But one wrong move...

You may get the same feelings when you indulge in a bad habit craving. At first it's thrilling and the rush is accompanied by a sense of control and mastery. But the balance is quickly upset when your body begins to call the shots and your craving turns into a physical addiction. Remember homeostasis: the body's natural tendency to maintain an internal stability? Cravings that become addictions prevent healthy homeostasis. You can bet that acrobat won't make it across the Falls under the influence. (Wait a minute, though, maybe gambling isn't such a good idea. We don't want to encourage a *new* risky habit! But you *do* get the point...)

To be happy and successful in a turbulent world, we all need to achieve a sense of balance and mastery. And nothing feels better than discovering the physical and mental clarity that emerges as you break your bad craving habit. It may take more than a day or a month, but soon you'll realize that you can have focus, concentration, and strength to face life's challenges without depending on an unhealthy relationship to a substance.

The Least You Need to Know

➤ Bad habits related to substances have both physical and emotional triggers and effects.

➤ Addiction is a serious outcome of a bad habit related to substances.

➤ You can learn to bring your life back into balance and to control your cravings.

➤ The challenge of breaking a bad habit craving is to take the responsibility for your pleasure away from the substance you're dependent on and reinvest it in yourself.

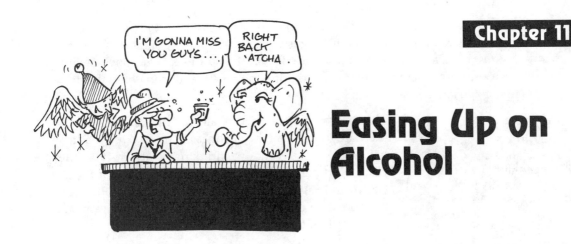

Chapter 11

Easing Up on Alcohol

In This Chapter

➤ Alcohol and the American lifestyle

➤ What alcohol does to your mind and body

➤ Choosing to abstain or moderate your drinking

➤ Establishing a healthy relationship with alcohol

Do you get tipsy from sipping a wine spritzer, while your best friend can belt down a couple of shots of tequila without feeling a thing? Neither one of you has a "problem" with alcohol—unless you can't *stop* drinking. Alcohol affects each individual in a unique way. The amount of alcohol *you* can handle—if any—depends on a variety of factors, including your family history, your current mood and general health, and personal circumstances.

Drinking: An American Pastime

Wake up this morning with a throbbing head and roiling stomach? Worried that something you said or did under the influence might come back to haunt you? If so, you're not alone. Far from it.

More than two-thirds of Americans drink, at least on occasion. We raise our glasses to toast to each other's health and good fortune. Our social lives often revolve around alcohol, at parties, business functions, sporting events, and bars. We have wine with meals and an after-dinner cognac. We drink to relax, to cheer up, to calm down, to become inspired, to escape, and simply because we enjoy the taste of liquor. Americans move at a fast pace, and a drink can take the edge off the pressures of keeping up with a cutting-edge society. That leads a lot of us to drink too much, and many of us down the slippery slope to *alcoholism*.

Strictly Speaking
Alcoholism is a chronic, progressive, potentially fatal disease characterized by physical dependence on alcohol, tolerance to its effects, and withdrawal symptoms when consumption is reduced or stopped.

Although each of us reacts to alcohol in a different way, there are some general guidelines about drinking that may help you evaluate your own drinking habits. In 1990, the U.S. Department of Agriculture and the U.S. Department of Health and Human Services defined moderate drinking as no more than one standard drink a day for most women and no more than two standard drinks a day for most men.

Just for the record, a standard drink is considered to be 12 ounces of beer, 5 ounces of wine, or 1.5 ounces of 80-proof distilled spirits. Each of these drinks contains roughly the same amount of absolute alcohol, approximately 0.5 ounces or 12 grams.

Presumably, then, anything more than 1 or 2 drinks a day is *immoderate* drinking, or drinking that has the potential to disrupt your health or personal life.

A New Angle
Until recently, drinking problems were largely a "man thing" with the vast majority of alcoholics being men. Today, equal rights has taken a dangerous turn: Women are catching up pretty quickly, and females now comprise about 43 percent of Alcoholics Anonymous members.

Alcohol and the Body 101

Ever wonder what's in that bottle of spirits that has the power to effect you so dramatically? The whirling dervish is ethyl alcohol (ethanol) and it occurs naturally from fermenting sugar and yeast.

As soon as you take a drink, 20 percent of the alcohol is immediately absorbed into the bloodstream through the stomach wall. The remaining 80 takes a little longer, because it goes through the small intestine first, but eventually gets to the bloodstream as well. Once on the move, alcohol travels throughout the body and affects almost every organ.

➤ **The Brain.** Alcohol slows down or depresses the brain's central control areas. Drowsiness, slowed reflexes, and uncoordination are the side-effects of moderate drinking (which is why drinking and driving is a deadly duo!). At the same time, however, alcohol also acts on the brain to loosen inhibitions, leading to feelings of relaxation, ease, and even animation. And there's the rub, right? It *feels* good.

➤ **The Liver.** While the liver is busy metabolizing 95 percent of the alcohol, it "forgets" other functions, such as maintaining adequate glucose (blood sugar) levels in the brain.

➤ **The Stomach.** Ever get a queasy feeling while drinking or afterward? Alcohol irritates the esophagus (windpipe) and the stomach. It causes the stomach to secrete digestive acids, which may trigger nausea, vomiting, and gastrointestinal bleeding.

➤ **The Kidneys.** Is the bathroom your best friend while you're drinking? Alcohol causes you to urinate more often and lose more fluids than you've just drunk, making you dehydrated.

➤ **The Mouth.** Do the words "dry mouth" mean anything to you? Overdrinking causes this unpleasant symptom because alcohol "confuses" the salivary glands, making the mouth dry up.

If you're like most people—and that's a big if considering how variable the effects of alcohol can be—the liver can metabolize approximately half an ounce to one ounce of pure alcohol per hour, which is the approximate content of a 12-ounce beer, a 5-ounce glass of wine, or a 1.5 ounce shot glass. If you drink more than that, you're more likely to become drunk and have a hangover the next day. Other factors that contribute to the way alcohol affects you include:

➤ **The total amount of alcohol you consume.** The more you drink, the "higher" you get, unless you drink *very* slowly.

➤ **Your size, gender, body build, and metabolism.** Generally speaking, the more you weigh, the more alcohol you can drink without becoming drunk; women don't metabolize alcohol as efficiently as men; and the quicker your body metabolizes food in general, the more efficiently it deals with alcohol, too.

➤ **The type and amount of food in your stomach.** If you drink on an empty stomach, alcohol will have a more immediate and greater effect. Dairy products slow alcohol's absorption by coating the stomach.

A New Angle

Didn't you always think that it was the difference in weight that made it possible for men to drink more than women? There's also a significant difference in the activity of an enzyme in the stomach tissue of males and females that breaks down alcohol before it reaches the bloodstream. This enzyme is four times more active in males than females. And women have proportionately more fat and less body water than men. Because alcohol is more soluble in water than in fat, it becomes more highly concentrated in a female's body.

To Drink, or Not to Drink, That Is the Question

Is the pleasure of drinking worth the unpleasant short-term side effects and the long-term health risks of drinking too much? While recent studies show that consuming one to two drinks daily significantly reduces the risk of heart disease in both men and women of all ages, that shouldn't become an excuse to drink more than your body—or your life—can handle.

Chronic, long-term drinking has many serious health risks. Hepatitis and cirrhosis (scarring) of the liver occurs as the liver goes on overload from a lifetime of processing alcohol through the body. Brain damage from excessive alcohol consumption is second only to Alzheimer's disease as a cause of memory loss and the deterioration of thinking skills in adults. Heavy alcohol use contributes to the risk of liver, stomach, colon, and breast cancer. Studies show that those one or two drinks a day can increase a woman's risk of breast cancer 30 to 50 percent!

If you still want to have a drink now and then, but you're afraid your drinking might be getting out of hand, it's important to do the work we described in Parts 1 and 2 of this book to discover why you're drinking. If you understand where the impulse to pick up that beer or down that scotch on the rocks comes from, you'll gain important clues about how to begin working to bring your drinking back to a level that's pleasurable and not damaging to your health, or to your relationships with other people.

Unfortunately, the properties of alcohol become progressively more lethal over time. And as your body builds a tolerance, you'll start to need more and more alcohol to achieve the same elusive feeling of pleasure and escape. If that urge for one drink too many is overtaking you, pause for a moment and consider where you could end up on this bad habit slippery slope. A brisk walk in the sunshine, hugging your child, going to the movies, or five minutes of deep breathing exercises to relax and calm yourself may be more productive alternatives to that drink you want so badly.

You may think this is funny, but we have one friend who's rarely ever imbibed alcohol in her life; whenever she's under stress, though, she blurts, "I could really use a drink right now." What does she do instead? She goes into a quiet room with no distractions and does ten minutes of yoga. It works for her every time. So it isn't the drink she really needs, it's the relief from stress that we've all learned to believe, in our society, having a drink supplies.

When Is Drinking a Problem?

Your relationship to alcohol is a very personal one, affecting your body in a very personal way. But the decision to drink or not to drink affects more than just you. Your work, your family, your friends, all of them become participants in your relationship with the bottle. Because when you're under the influence, your whole life goes under the influence as well.

Answer these questions to find some clues about whether your drinking is becoming a problem:

1. Do you ever drink to get drunk?
   *Yes*____   *No*____

2. Do you think drinking will help solve your problems?
   *Yes*____   *No*____

3. Do you drink to calm down before an upcoming stressful situation?
   *Yes*____   *No*____

4. When you drink, do you experience a mood change, becoming more aggressive or more depressed?
   *Yes*____   *No*____

5. Do you ever worry about where and when you'll drink next?
   *Yes*____   *No*____

6. Do you experience frequent hangovers or blackouts?
   *Yes*____   *No*____

7. Do you ever lie about drinking?
   *Yes*____   *No*____

8. Have you ever missed work or other appointments because of drinking?
   *Yes*____   *No*____

9. Do you often drink alone?
   *Yes*____   *No*____

10. Do you sometimes crave a drink in the morning?
    *Yes*____   *No*____

109

If you answered "yes" to two or more of the preceding questions, you may be becoming dependent on alcohol. You certainly need to seriously question your drinking habits and consider how you can learn to better control your behavior in this regard.

Too Much at the Holiday Party...Again

Because alcohol tends to loosen up your inhibitions, it seems a perfect "socializer" for people who feel anxious at parties or other social situations.

Unfortunately, when you loosen up too much with alcohol, it often causes more than a hangover. Overdrinking at an office party or during a date can have unpleasant, even dangerous consequences. Telling off the boss, flirting outrageously with a colleague, revealing too much personal information about yourself, or falling down in front of the company president are just a few of the ways that losing control can affect your judgment—as well as your professional reputation.

If you can, avoid alcoholic beverages altogether at these functions. If you can't do that—or don't want to—have one drink and then switch to ginger ale or sparkling water. And who says you have to announce that your beverage is nonalcoholic? Only your bartender needs to know. If you need more discipline than this to control drinking at a party or social function, go with a friend and make a deal about the limits you'd like to set for your drinking. Agree on a time to stop and a time to leave the party, maybe making plans to go to a movie or meet someone afterwards—so you're not there at 1 a.m. when the only people who're still partying are the ones who've had too much to drink.

Interestingly, it may well be possible to be in a social situation, and yet be drinking alone. For example, if you come home after work, plop yourself down, and pick up a drink instead of communicating with your spouse and playing with your kids, you're drinking alone, even though you're surrounded by people.

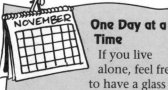

One Day at a Time

If you live alone, feel free to have a glass of wine with dinner or an occasional cocktail at the end of your day—if you can handle it. But it's important to keep careful control over how much you drink, and why you're drinking. Set limits and stick to them, or remove all alcohol from the house.

Drinking Alone

Overdrinking is a problem no matter where you are, at a big party with hundreds of guests or alone in your own living room. However, one sign that you've lost control of your drinking, or that you're drinking to mask feelings of loneliness or anxiety, is drinking more than you plan to, by yourself, on a regular basis.

Drinking alone can be a very unhealthy way to protect yourself from feelings of loneliness and insecurity. Indulging in this bad habit will only prevent you from facing, and then overcoming, your difficulties with connecting to other people. If you're worried about how much you drink when you're by yourself, ask a trusted friend or health professional for advice.

Hung Over and Hating It

"I feel sorry for people who don't drink," said notorious alcoholic Dean Martin. "When they wake up in the morning, that's as good as they're going to feel all day." Brave—and perhaps foolish—words for a man who died of liver disease!

A hangover is your body's way of telling you that you've poisoned yourself with alcohol, and you'll feel pretty crummy until your body recovers. Here are some of the reasons why your body reacts in such an unpleasant way:

➤ **Production of acetaldehyde.** Ever heard of formaldehyde, the substance morticians use to preserve corpses? Well, your liver produces a related chemical when it breaks down ethanol (the active part of alcohol).

➤ **Dehydration.** Alcohol is a diuretic, which means it causes your kidneys to excrete more fluids as they remove alcohol from the body. Dehydration makes you feel weak and lethargic, and dries out your mouth like there's no tomorrow.

➤ **Toxic chemicals.** Produced during the fermentation and distillation process, certain chemicals called congeners can mildly poison you if you drink too much.

➤ **Effects on sleep.** Isn't it strange that you can pass out big time and yet wake up exhausted? The anesthetic effect of alcohol interferes with the brain's ability to produce an adequate amount of REM (the dreaming portion of sleep), which partially accounts for the morning fatigue you may feel after you've overindulged.

Sober Is Better

If you're reading this chapter, gaining control over your drinking may be sounding good to you. Maybe your drinking is limiting your social life. If you're spending most of your free evenings at a local bar, it's unlikely you get out to the theater, a gallery opening, or a poetry reading very often. And what about exercise? It sure is tough to hang on to a martini while pumping iron.

If you watch *Cheers* reruns lately and shout at Norm and Cliff to "get a life," chances are you're already looking for other things to do with yourself besides have a drink.

Cold Turkey
NEVER drink if you're:

➤ Pregnant or trying to conceive

➤ Driving or operating heavy machinery

➤ Taking medication, including over-the-counter drugs

➤ Recovering from alcohol addiction

➤ Under 21

Choosing Not to Drink

There are many good reasons to abstain from drinking alcohol altogether. If you have a family history of alcoholism, medical problems that contraindicate the use of alcohol, or simply do not enjoy the way drinking makes you feel during and after an episode with the bottle, then you have very good reasons to choose this option.

Depending on how heavily you've been drinking in recent months, it may be difficult to stop on your own, without the guidance of a doctor or other health professional. We suggest you make an appointment with a physician to work out a plan that's best for you.

Learning Moderation

If you decide to drink moderately and responsibly, here are some tips—several of them from the National Institute on Alcohol Abuse and Alcoholism—to help get you started:

➤ **Keep track of your drinking.** Oh, yes indeed, you're going to need your Daily Habit Log as you come to terms with your drinking. Note when you feel the urge to drink and what triggers it, how much you drink and what it feels like, and the after-effects your drinking episode creates.

➤ **Set a drinking goal.** Choose a limit—daily, weekly, or for a special event. Stick to it. If you can't, that's a sign you might need some outside help.

➤ **Designate yourself the "designated driver."** If you feel at all uncomfortable about turning down a drink, let your friends know that you're driving yourself home—sober.

➤ **Bring your own non-alcoholic beverages.**

➤ **Drink slowly.** Sip your drink, preferably making it last at least an hour. Then take a break of one hour before you have another drink (if you choose). In between, drink plenty of water and fruit juice, which will help flush your system.

➤ **Take a break from alcohol.** Pick a day or two—or more—when you won't drink at all. Then, try to stop drinking for a week. Think about how you feel, physically and emotionally, on the days you abstain. We guarantee you'll feel more alert and energetic. Soon you may choose not to drink at all.

Cold Turkey
If you've been a heavy drinker in recent months, cutting out all alcohol may produce withdrawal symptoms, including nausea, diarrhea, increase in blood pressure, shakiness, weakness, and insomnia. If your symptoms are severe, make an appointment with your doctor as soon as possible.

➤ **Learn how to say no.** Remember what we said in Chapter 10: Gaining control over your bad habit gives you *more* choices, not fewer. You are *not* required to drink when people around you are drinking. You do not have to take a drink that some-one hands you.

➤ **Expand your horizons.** Find something new to do with the time you used to spend drinking or hung-over. Eat out more often, go to the movies, take an adult-education class, learn a new sport, or join the gym. Depending on how much you used to drink, you may be able to afford these new ventures with the money you're saving by skipping the alcohol.

➤ **Get support.** We know it and you know it: Cutting down on your drinking won't be easy. Ask your friends and family to help you in reaching your goals. And if your "friends" don't support your decision, it may be time to find some new associates. Talk to your doctor. Join a support group (see Chapter 24 for more advice).

➤ **Guard against temptations.** Avoid people, places, or situations that trigger the urge to overindulge. If you know that your friend Bob doesn't know the meaning of the phrase, "I'll just have a club soda, thanks," on a Friday night, choose to see him at times he—and you—will be less likely to drink.

➤ **Watch your mood.** Don't drink when you're angry, upset, or depressed. Strong emotions like these are common triggers of drinking.

➤ **Monitor your condition.** Some people can *never* drink because they are unable to tolerate the effects of drinking or to control how much they drink. If you suspect you are one of these people, talk to your doctor or another health professional.

➤ **Don't give up.** Slow but steady wins this race. Whether your goal is to abstain completely or cut down to moderation, take it one day at a time.

The Least You Need to Know

➤ Alcohol is the most commonly used drug in the United States.

➤ Alcohol affects every organ system in the body, including the brain, stomach, and liver.

➤ It's important to weigh the risks and benefits of your drinking habits on a regular basis.

➤ There are several effective methods of reducing or eliminating drinking.

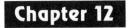

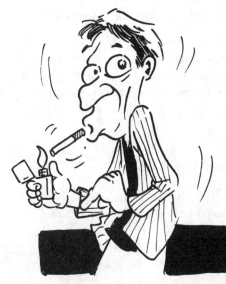

Put That Thing Out!

In This Chapter

➤ Creating the profile of a smoker

➤ How nicotine gets you hooked

➤ Learning to stop, for good

➤ Your smoke-free future

"It'd be like losing my hand."

"I've tried. God knows I've tried. I just don't have the willpower. Smoking is part of my life."

"Quit smoking? Never. I like living on the edge and to hell with people who tell me I should quit."

Do any of these statements sound familiar to you? Do you feel that your smoking habit is so entrenched that you'd never be able to live without it? Have you tried before and failed? Or are you digging in your heels and refusing to heed the best advice from family and friends (as well as medical experts around the world)? The problem is that, unlike many other bad habits, there's no way to moderate a cigarette habit. You really can't have just one or two cigarettes. You can't taper down and control your habit. You might just get down to one or two a day, for a week or so of white-knuckle effort. Soon you're back up to a half a pack, a pack, or more a day.

You're not alone in your struggle. More than 46 million Americans continue to smoke, even though they know—as you do—the dire health risks involved. Does that mean you and your fellow smokers are too weak and lacking in willpower? Hardly. You're fighting a very tough battle against the extremely addictive substance of nicotine, as well as against years of learned behaviors related to smoking.

Why, Oh Why, Is Quitting Smoking So Hard?

There's no doubt about it: Quitting smoking is one of the toughest challenges known to woman or man. The American Lung Association estimates that nearly 30 percent of smokers try to quit each year, but only two to three percent make it. The average smoker tries to quit four times before being successful. Yet half of all living Americans who've ever smoked have managed to quit. And you can, too—for your health, for your sense of self-esteem and self-control, for your future.

Nicotine: Is It Addictive?

The answer to that question is an undeniable and resounding YES. Former U.S. Surgeon General C. Everett Koop compares nicotine's grip on its users to that of heroin. According to a study performed at the Henry Ford Health Sciences Center in Detroit, about 90 percent of smokers are persistent daily users and 10 percent are occasional users. That's almost the exact reverse of another bad habit, excessive drinking. Only 10 to 15 percent of people who drink become dependent, problem drinkers, while most people use alcohol on an occasional basis.

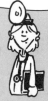

Strictly Speaking
Nicotine is a colorless, quick-acting poison in cigarette smoke. Nicotine is also used to kill insects in farming and to fight parasites in veterinary medicine.

What makes nicotine so addictive? Just 11 seconds after you take a puff of a cigarette—within five heartbeats—nicotine reaches the brain, where it attaches itself to certain receptors in a part of the brain called the limbic system. This action releases chemicals called neurotransmitters that affect cognition and alertness, as well as feelings of pleasure and satisfaction. Nicotine also increases the brain's uptake of glucose, an energy nutrient. Finally, nicotine slows down communication between certain parts of the brain, which causes you to feel more relaxed. Nicotine also causes your heart rate and blood pressure to rise, giving you a sense of stimulation and increased energy.

Now you can see why you crave nicotine: It helps you think faster, calm down, and feel pleasure—all within 11 seconds. If you smoke a pack a day and take 10 puffs from each cigarette, you stimulate your brain with nicotine 200 times a day. Unfortunately, though, you'll probably need more and more nicotine to get the same effect because most people develop a nicotine tolerance.

And those are just the purely physiological aspects of cigarette addiction. There's more, much more, to this habit than meets the lungs and brain.

The Very Feel of It

French existentialist philosopher Jean-Paul Sartre, a lifelong smoker who finally quit, wrote, "In truth, I did not much care for the taste of tobacco that I was going to lose. Rather, it was the meaning of the act of smoking. I used to smoke at performances, mornings at work, evenings after dinner, and it seemed to me that in ceasing to smoke, I was going to subtract some of the interest of the performance, some of the evening dinner's savor, some of the fresh vivacity of the morning's work."

Like Sartre, you've probably become accustomed to associating cigarettes with certain activities—having your morning coffee, writing your sales reports, taking a break from the kids. Not only does the sensation nicotine provides help you through your day, but now you're used to the feel of the cigarette in your hand and mouth, the sound of the match as it bursts into flame, the way you play with the ashtray as you smoke.

And then there are some added habitual pleasures. Maybe you enjoy the few extra moments that lighting a cigarette takes up during a conversation (or confrontation). Or maybe it's the seductive sense of intimacy when a stranger lights your cigarette (ever seen Bette Davis in *Now, Voyager*?). In the theater, these activities are called "business," the busy-ness that distracts from the subject at hand. For the employee bawled out by the boss, smoking reassures. For an insecure person seeking companionship, smoking bolsters confidence. For the harried parent, smoking is an escape.

What Smoking Does to Your Body

Scientists have identified more than 43 different substances in tobacco that cause cancer. Altogether, cigarette smoke contains about 4,000 chemicals, including trace amounts of such known poisons as DDT, arsenic, and formaldehyde.

Here's how the nicotine and other chemicals in cigarette smoke affect the various systems in your body:

Circulation: Nicotine triggers the release of certain hormones that act to constrict blood vessels, impairing circulation to the body's extremities and raising blood pressure 10 to 15 percent. This rise in blood pressure increases the risk of stroke and heart attack.

Blood: Carbon monoxide in cigarette smoke replaces up to 12 percent of the oxygen normally carried by red blood cells, robbing your tissues of oxygen. Physical activity becomes more strenuous.

Lungs: Smoking stunts the growth of teens' lungs and decreases breathing capacity. Tar in cigarette smoke coats and kills lung tissue. Later in life, this may lead to lung cancer or emphysema—a lung disease that destroys the walls of the lungs' air sacs.

A New Angle

Once men outnumbered women when it came to lung cancer, but now the tide is turning. In 1987, lung cancer surpassed breast cancer as the leading cause of cancer deaths among women. This rising rate is expected to peak around the year 2010. And it isn't the only cancer risk smoking increases for women: Women who smoke are at far greater risk for cervical cancer. If you're a woman smoker, make sure you get an annual Pap smear and see your gynecologist every six months. Cervical cancer is curable if caught early—but deadly if it's not.

Heart: Smoking makes the heart work harder to pump an extra 10 to 25 times per minute. In addition, less oxygen reaches the heart from the damaged lungs and carbon dioxide-filled blood, which may cause heart disease.

Skin: Smoking destroys elastin, the elastic fibers that keep skin smooth and wrinkle-free. Nicotine in cigarette smoke also constricts blood vessels near the skin's surface, so less oxygen and moisture reach the tissue.

Eyes: According to new research, smokers are twice as likely to develop macular degeneration, or damage to the center of the retina.

Teeth: The tar in cigarettes turns teeth yellow, and smoking inhibits the activity of antibodies that protect your gums from periodontal disease. Smokers are nearly twice as likely to suffer tooth loss than nonsmokers: Tooth decay and gum disease are also more prevalent among smokers.

Mouth, throat, and voice box: These delicate tissues are exposed repetitively to the cancer-causing agents of tobacco smoke. Mouth and esophageal cancer is the result.

Stomach: Cigarette smoke stimulates overproduction of the stomach's gastric juices, which can cause or exacerbate ulcers and other gastrointestinal problems.

Smoking Stats and Your Health

All right. We know we're hitting hard in this chapter, but we want to arm you with as many statistics as possible to firm up your resolve to quit. The facts about smoking might just take your breath away....

➤ Tobacco use remains the leading preventable cause of death in the United States, causing more than 400,000 deaths each year and resulting in an annual cost of more than $50 billion in direct medical expenses.

➤ Each year, smoking kills more people than AIDS, alcohol, drug abuse, car crashes, murders, suicides, and fires—combined.

➤ Nationally, smoking results in more than five million years of potential life lost each year.

➤ More than five million children alive today will die prematurely because of decisions they make as adolescents.

➤ A smoker's fetus or infant has a 25 to 50 percent higher death rate than that of a nonsmoking mother.

Cold Turkey
Second-hand smoke is no joke! In 1993, the U.S. Environmental Protection Agency found that fumes given off from the tips of lighted cigarettes have higher concentrations of cancer-causing chemicals than the smoke that smokers inhale. If you stop smoking, then you may be saving other lives along with your own. Avoid smoking around infants and young children especially.

The Good News About Quitting

Okay, enough already. It's time to look at the healthy future you have in store when you decide to quit smoking once and for all:

Within 12 hours: Your body begins to heal quickly after your last puff of a cigarette. The levels of carbon monoxide and nicotine in your system decline, and your heart and lungs begin to repair themselves.

Within 24 hours: Your chances of having a heart attack decrease.

Within 48 hours: Your sense of smell and taste is returning. Your lung function begins to improve. You may be coughing more than usual as your body rejects the toxins in your lungs.

One Day at a Time
Think of the short-term benefits of not smoking. You don't have to leave the room (or the building). You don't have to find a match. You don't end up with that yucky taste in your mouth. By thinking of the "small" benefits instead of the longer-term, and more serious risks, you might be able to resist the immediate gratification that comes with a puff on a cigarette.

119

Within three months: Your circulation improves, as does your aerobic capacity. You'll feel less winded, and exercise will become much easier to perform.

Within nine months: You'll be coughing much less, and any previous shortness of breath will dissipate. Your immune system also improves, and you're likely to suffer fewer colds.

Within one year: Your risk of heart disease will be half that of a smoker. Half.

Within five years: You'll cut in half your risks for lung, mouth, and throat cancer. Stroke and heart disease risk approaches that of a nonsmoker.

Within 10 years: Your chance of developing lung cancer matches that of a nonsmoker.

Within 15 years: Your risk of dying from a smoking-related disease is the same as for someone who's never smoked.

The benefits of quitting smoking are amazing—so amazing we don't think you'll need to do a "risk-benefit" analysis for this particular habit. There really isn't a good enough reason to keep pumping these poisons through your body. Your body will learn to live and thrive without nicotine, and so will your mind and emotions.

"Sure I Can Quit Smoking, I Do It All the Time"

Cold turkey—stopping smoking altogether, all at once—is, for most people, the only way to go. Tapering off the number of cigarettes you smoke simply doesn't work in most cases, because it allows the smoker to continue to put off the inevitable, usually forever. (Please note, however, that we mean "cold turkey" only in relation to cigarettes. The use of the nicotine patch, which we discuss later, is a way to "taper off" *without* cigarettes.) The one exception to this rule is if you are a very heavy smoker—two packs or more a day. In that case, you may want to decrease your smoking a few cigarettes a day until you're at a pack a day. And then go cold turkey. Here's how to do it:

➤ **Choose to quit for yourself.** We know the pressure to quit is probably coming at you from all sides—your spouse, your mother, your friends, your doctor. But your attempt to quit won't be successful unless YOU really want to change.

➤ **List your reasons to quit and keep them close.** It's important to remember why you want to stop smoking: Your short-term and your long-term goals. Create a Ladder of Success like the one described in Chapter 8 and post it on your bulletin board to remind you of what you'll be gaining by losing the smoking habit.

➤ **Set a start date.** The Great American Smoke-Out, your birthday, next Thursday: Choose a date that has meaning for you and that's far enough in advance to allow you to prepare your environment. Don't make it too far in advance or you might lose your resolve.

➤ **Prepare your environment.** Clear out all smoking paraphernalia. Empty your house and office of lighters, ashtrays, and cigarettes—all of them. Launder your clothes and even your upholstery to remove that stale tobacco odor that could trigger the urge to smoke.

➤ **Maintain your Daily Habit Log.** Record each time you smoke or have the urge to smoke. Don't empty your ashtrays until you've counted how many you've smoked and written that number down. Becoming aware of why you want a cigarette will help you replace it with more healthful alternatives. If you smoke to relieve stress, perform deep breathing exercises or meditate instead. If you smoke for energy, take a walk or talk to a perky loved one.

➤ **Keep track of the benefits.** Does your mouth feel fresher? Are your teeth getting whiter? Was it easier to climb that second flight of stairs? Write it down, remember it, and keep adding to the list of pleasant side effects.

➤ **Avoid triggers.** What makes you want to smoke most? Once you find that out, try to avoid the stimuli as much as possible. Switch to tea if the taste of coffee makes you want to smoke. Go to a smoke-free restaurant instead of a bar if seeing other people smoke triggers a craving, etc.

➤ **Deal with side effects.** There's no doubt about it: You're going to feel some pretty icky side effects as you withdraw from cigarettes. Here are a few of the most common and some ideas to combat them.

Smoking Withdrawal Side Effects	What to Do About Them
Constipation	Eat more roughage, such as raw fruit, vegetables, and whole grain cereals. Drink six to eight glasses of water a day. Get plenty of exercise.
Dry Mouth	Sip ice-cold water or chew sugarless gum.
Fatigue	Nap if you need to until your body heals and returns to vitality. Deep breathing exercises, which bring oxygen to the brain, will also help make you more alert.
Headaches	Take a warm bath or shower. Try relaxation or meditation techniques.
Hunger	Eat vegetables and fruit and drink low-calorie liquids.

continues

continued

Smoking Withdrawal Side Effects	What to Do About Them
Insomnia	Cut out caffeine, especially after 6 p.m. Try deep breathing exercises just before you go to bed.
Sore throat, sore gums, or sore tongue	Sip water or chew gum.
Tension	Exercise is the very best remedy for the sense of pent-up stress and tension that often accompanies nicotine withdrawal.

➤ **Occupy your hands and mouth.** Fill a "goody bag" with nutritious alternatives: sugarless gum, mints, toothpicks, water, anything (healthy) that'll keep your mouth and your mind busy.

➤ **Get support.** Ask your spouse or a friend to quit with you. Tell family and friends you're quitting—but set a limit on the nagging or "encouraging" they're allowed to do.

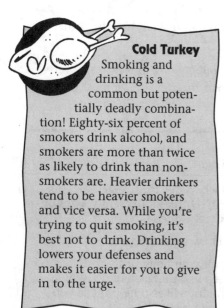

Cold Turkey

Smoking and drinking is a common but potentially deadly combination! Eighty-six percent of smokers drink alcohol, and smokers are more than twice as likely to drink than non-smokers are. Heavier drinkers tend to be heavier smokers and vice versa. While you're trying to quit smoking, it's best not to drink. Drinking lowers your defenses and makes it easier for you to give in to the urge.

➤ **Join a stop-smoking program.** The American Heart Association and the American Lung Association offer a variety of programs designed to support you in your healthy goal.

➤ **Plan to spend what you'll save.** Give yourself financial incentives and disincentives. Make a list of things you'd like to buy for yourself or someone else with your "profits"—the money you won't be spending on cigarettes.

➤ **Change your eating habits.** Drinking alcohol and coffee may trigger the need to smoke, so you may want to cut back. Drink milk or juice instead. As your taste buds return to life, experiment with eating new foods and trying different cuisines.

➤ **Create obstacles.** You can't smoke when you're wet, so take up swimming or other kinds of exercise. Knitting, needlework, crossword puzzles, and cooking use your hands so much that it's harder to smoke.

➤ **Practice deep breathing.** Breathe slowly through the nose into the stomach, lungs, and upper chest, and then slowly exhale until your upper chest, lungs, and stomach are empty of air. This helps relax you and bring you back into balance by pumping oxygen to the brain through the blood.

➤ **Never allow yourself "just one," and never give up.** Saying "I'll just have this one cigarette to get me through," may be tempting, but such an approach is sure to backfire. Know this: It's almost impossible to have "just one" cigarette. At the same time, if you "fall off the wagon," don't give up. Dust yourself off, and try again.

Hair of the Dog, Smoke-wise

A variety of new products, now available over-the-counter as well as by prescription, can help you beat the smoking habit by providing your body with a steady dose of nicotine. Nicotine replacement therapy (NRT) now comes in three forms: patches and gums, available over-the-counter, and nasal sprays, available only by prescription. *Progressive Grocer* magazine estimated in April 1997 that over-the-counter smoking cessation is now a $300 million business.

It may seem odd to provide yourself doses of the very drug you're trying to stop using, but studies have shown that nicotine replacement will help you stop smoking for good. When measured against a placebo, nicotine replacement therapy has nearly doubled the initial quitting rate and doubled the number who remain abstinent six months or one year later, especially when combined with behavior modification therapy. Counseling can teach smokers how to break their associations with cigarettes and how to find effective substitutes for the benefits they derived from smoking, including relaxation, mental stimulation, and weight control—plus the other methods we suggested earlier in the chapter.

NRT works by curbing the discomforts of withdrawal without providing the rapid, higher doses of nicotine that directly affect the brain. And it does so without exposing you—and the people around you—to the harmful ingredients in cigarette smoke—the tar and other carcinogens in tobacco.

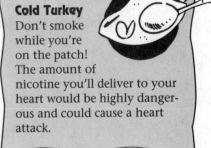

Cold Turkey
Don't smoke while you're on the patch! The amount of nicotine you'll deliver to your heart would be highly dangerous and could cause a heart attack.

Nicotine patches deliver a measured dose of nicotine to the bloodstream through the skin. Slowly, over the course of several weeks, the dose of nicotine is lowered, gradually reducing your need for it. You place one patch, which contains one of several different doses of nicotine depending on your needs, on your upper body every day. The usual course of treatment for NRT is about six to eight weeks. Ask your doctor or pharmacist for more advice.

Nicotine gum also delivers a dose of nicotine to the bloodstream and allows you to taper the amount of the drug you receive over a course of time. Some smokers prefer using NRT in gum form because chewing allows them to use their mouths and helps to reduce the craving for a cigarette. Treatment continues for three to four months.

Nicotine nasal spray is a new treatment that tends to deliver nicotine to the brain more quickly than the other methods. At this time, the nasal spray is available only by prescription, and is used for about the same length of time and in the same intervals as nicotine gum.

Take a Deep Breath

It's tough, it's tedious, it's frustrating. But try to stay motivated by thinking of quitting smoking as a precious gift you're giving to yourself—the gift of a healthier body, a clearer mind, a longer life, a new sense of confidence and self control. Take this opportunity to start being kind to yourself. Nurture your interests and your strengths. You're going to have a longer and healthier life ahead of you, and now is the time to learn to take advantage of it! Breathe in that fresh air and feel your strong heart and lungs move with the rhythm of life. Breathe out: Ahhhhhhhhhhh....

The Least You Need to Know

➤ Nicotine is a very addictive drug, and smoking is one of the hardest habits to break.

➤ There's not one single good reason to start smoking, and every reason to make the effort to stop.

➤ Behavior modification techniques, such as rewarding yourself for your efforts and finding healthier substitutes for smoking, can help you break the cigarette habit.

➤ Your health and vitality return over time after you stop smoking.

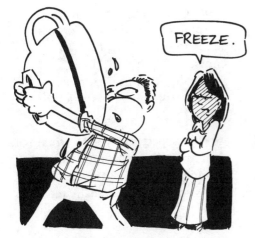

FREEZE.

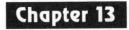

Chapter 13

Calming the Caffeine Jitters

In This Chapter

➤ Life in the "fast" lane

➤ What caffeine does to your mind and body

➤ Controlling your caffeine intake

➤ Energy from a new source

Ah, caffeine, the most widely used drug in the world. How we love it. America in the twenty-first century moves at the speed of light. Between working, taking care of the house and the kids, checking in on our parents, and just plain getting things done, we simply exhaust ourselves. For many of us, caffeine equals energy and we'll take as much as we can get.

Running on Empty: When Only a Jolt Will Do

Can't get through the morning without your coffee? Need a piece of chocolate in the afternoon to get through that slump? You're far from the only one. In the United States alone, more than 80 percent of adults consume caffeine on a regular (shall we say, habitual?) basis, and, on average, ingest the equivalent of about three cups of coffee a day (about 280 milligrams). A choice few of us (about 20 percent) have really got it bad, consuming up to 500 mg or more.

As ubiquitous as caffeine is (Did you ever think there would be as many Starbucks as Gaps?), it's a drug that produces intense effects on the human mind and body. For most people, the effects are pleasurable. But for others, a little too much caffeine leads to fragmented concentration, headaches, heartburn, insomnia, irritability, shakiness, and chronic gastrointestinal problems. The good news: In moderate amounts (Yes, moderation. What a concept!), caffeine poses no health or emotional risks, either in the long- or short-term.

On the other hand, you're probably reading this because you suspect that you're drinking too much caffeine. If so, you'll be happy to know that you can find the energy you need from more healthful sources, and you can break your caffeine habit without too much trouble. When you do, you'll be amazed to discover that less caffeine can actually mean *more* energy!

Caffeine and Your Body: Welcome to Central Perk

Caffeine is a *stimulant*, a member of a group of alkaloids called xanthine derivatives. Other xanthine derivatives include theophylline and theobromine. All three act to speed up your central nervous system. Coffee contains only caffeine, but other substances contain small amounts of theophylline and theobromine as well.

Within 15 minutes after you consume caffeine, the drug begins to take effect. It acts primarily to increase the amount of two essential hormones: epinephrine (also known as adrenaline) and cortisol. The hormones act together to trigger the following biological events:

Strictly Speaking
A **stimulant** is any substance that speeds up the body's activities. Caffeine belongs to a family of stimulants found in plants called xanthine derivatives.

➤ An increase of heart rate and blood pressure.

➤ An increase in respiration rate (because caffeine also relaxes smooth muscle tissues such as those that line the bronchial tubes).

➤ An increase in production of stomach acid.

➤ An increase in urinary output.

➤ Stimulation of brain activity.

The effect caffeine produces varies considerably from person to person, but most people feel more alert and better able to concentrate after they've had a cup of coffee or tea. This pleasant effect can last for an hour or two—just enough to get you going if you need a little physical encouragement.

But as you know too well, too much caffeine can cause some pretty nasty side effects that distract and disturb us as much as—or more than—any ordinary dip in energy. David Lettermen devoted one of his "Top Ten Lists" to the effects of caffeine excess. Our favorite of his "Signs that you've had too much coffee" include:

> "When you call radio talk shows, they ask you to turn *yourself* down."

> "Last time you got a good night's sleep, Madonna was a virgin."

> "You're up to four heart attacks a day."

As amusing as these tidbits might be, they illustrate the side effects of consuming too much caffeine very well. In short, when it comes to caffeine, too much of a good thing is a bad thing.

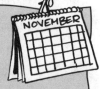

Cold Turkey
Chronic over-use of caffeinated products may be a way of self-medicating for clinical depression or an anxiety disorder. If you're concerned about that you may have some deeper, unresolved issues, talk to your doctor as soon as you can. There are much more effective, and less physically disruptive medications and therapies available.

How Less Caffeine Equals More Energy

Virtually all caffeine is eliminated from the body 12 to 24 hours after it was last consumed, taking with it all its effects and side effects. And that's what keeps you going back for more: You crave it! Think of it: Coffee's become so synonymous with energy and productivity that one of the hottest new Internet software programs is called Java. For a little more than a buck, you can drink a great caffe latte or down a liter of ice-cold soda and get a boost without much effort. Forget about exercising, meditation, deep breathing, and developing good time management skills!

Caffeine may give you a quick fix, but it can't replace the healthy benefits of taking care of your body and your mind. Couch potatoes with non-existent fitness levels aren't going to match the energy of someone who works out three times a week just by ingesting caffeine. Sustained mental concentration and focus aren't yours through the magic of caffeine. (How many walls did you walk into today?) A dose of caffeine pales beside the energy that comes from getting more oxygen to the blood and brain by practicing yoga or deep-breathing exercises. As for time management, what you need most may be a daily organizer, not another caffeinated beverage.

One Day at a Time
To ensure a good night's sleep, avoid all caffeine products at least 3.5 hours before you go to bed. If you still have insomnia, avoid caffeine after dinner or lunch. If you're highly sensitive, you may have to cut out all caffeine from your diet in order to sleep well.

"Okay," you say, "I get it. But while I'm working on all this other stuff, what do I do about caffeine?" Here are the first things you'll need to do to control your caffeine habit:

➤ Figure out how much caffeine you consume on a daily basis.

➤ Figure out what level of caffeine consumption triggers more productivity and health losses than gains. Learn to know your limit.

Caffeine Here, There, Everywhere

Where does this high-octane elixir come from? Caffeine is a naturally occurring substance found in the leaves, seeds, or fruits of more than 60 different plants. The most famous caffeinated plants are coffee and cocoa beans, kola nuts, and tea leaves. Caffeine is also an active ingredient in many medications.

The following statistics, provided by the National Coffee Association, National Soft Drink Association, the Tea Council of the United States, and the FDA's Center for Drugs and Biologics reveal the caffeine content of common products.

Get that Mo-Jo Working

By far, most Americans derive the lion's share of their caffeine by drinking that cup of Joe. You might be surprised at the wide range of caffeine levels that exists, depending on the type of bean and the processing method used.

Caffeine Levels in Coffee

Type of Coffee	Caffeine Content (6 oz)
Decaffeinated	2–5 mg
Instant	60–100 mg
Drip or brewed	80–175 mg
Espresso	60–120 mg
Cappuccino	60–120 mg
Coffee ice cream	58 mg (1 cup)

Although we tend to think of espresso as the strongest coffee, isn't it interesting that it actually has *less* caffeine that regular "American" coffee?

"Don't Tell Me to Drink Tea..."

"A cup of tea will never be a cup of coffee," you say. "Tea is for wimps. And herbal tea? What're you *nuts*?" We'll agree with you on the first point. But if you're looking to reduce your consumption of caffeine and you can't just drink one cup of coffee, you might want to give tea a second look. Tea generally has less caffeine than coffee, so you might be able to drink more of it each day and still reduce your daily caffeine intake.

Caffeine Levels in Tea

Type of Tea	Caffeine Content (8 oz)
Black tea	50–100 mg (depending on time brewed)
Lemon ginseng tea	50 mg
Green Tea	8–30 mg (depending on time brewed)
Snapple Iced Tea	25 mg
Arizona Iced Tea	20 mg

For the health conscious, consider that green tea, with it's very low caffeine levels, is also under study as an anti-cancer agent. In general, tea (of whatever variety) is the most-consumed beverage worldwide and is linked to a lower risk of heart disease and cancer.

As for coffee's healthful benefits: The aromatic steam that rises from a fresh, hot cup contains antioxidants that when inhaled may produce a healthy effect. But once the Joe goes cold, you're out of luck.

Bring on the Bubbly

Sodas of all types, including a few of the benign-looking light-colored, fruity-tasting types, can really pack a caffeine punch. Make sure you check the labels before you imbibe. Look for the sugar content, too. The sugar-caffeine connection is one you might want to learn to avoid. And if some sodas give you stomachaches when you drink too much, consider this: Mechanics often recommend using cola to clean off gunk that accumulates on your car's battery.

Caffeine Levels in Soft Drinks

Soft Drink	Caffeine Content (12 oz)
Mountain Dew	55 mg
Coca-Cola	46.8 mg

continues

continued

Soft Drink	Caffeine Content (12 oz)
Sunkist orange soda	40 mg
Diet Pepsi	36 mg

How Sweet It Is

You probably think that chocolate rush comes from sugar alone, right? Guess again. It's the sugar-caffeine connection.

Caffeine Levels in Chocolate

Type of Chocolate	Amount	Caffeine Content
Hot Chocolate	8 oz	3–32 mg
Milk chocolate	1 oz	1–15 mg
Dark chocolate	1 oz	5–35 mg
Baker's chocolate	1 oz	26 mg

Water? Caffeinated Water?

You bet. Some genius combined two current trends—one for spring water and the other for caffeine—and the result is sure to keep you shaking!

Caffeine Levels in Caffeinated Water

Brand	Caffeine Content (half liter)
Edge 20	145 mg
Java Water	125 mg
Krank 20	100 mg
Aqua Blast	90 mg
Water Joe	70 mg

We don't want to seem old-fashioned, but we strongly recommend you drink at least eight glasses of pure, *uncaffeinated* water or fruit juice daily. Leave caffeine out of your water supply.

Taking What's Good for You

Throughout history, caffeine has been used as a medicine. During the 1500s, Europeans used caffeinated beverages to treat headaches, coughs, and vertigo. In recent years, caffeine has been used as a highly successful treatment for migraines. But you might be surprised at how many different kinds of medications contain caffeine.

In the United States, the Food and Drug Administration regulates the use of caffeine in over-the-counter medications and requires manufacturers to list caffeine as an active ingredient on each product's label. If you're highly sensitive to caffeine's effects, pay close attention to the ingredients in the drugs you take. Caffeine is found in something as common as Excedrin (65 mg) or Midol (32 mg).

A New Angle

Believe it or not, decaffeinated coffees and teas are NOT completely free of caffeine. The decaffeination process only removes 97 percent of the caffeine, leaving about 2 to 5 mg in each cup.

Just One Cup Won't Hurt—Will It?

Okay, so now you know how much caffeine is in the stuff you eat and drink. You've figured out how much you consume every day. Let's take a look at where the experts place the caffeine "edge."

Considering how many of us love the stuff, it's a good thing caffeine is a fairly benign substance. Study after study shows that in moderate amounts—under about 650 mg a day, and preferably under 300 mg a day—caffeine poses no health risks whatsoever. In moderate amounts, caffeine doesn't cause cancer or heart disease or ulcers. And although you can become dependent on caffeine, it isn't in the same category as other drugs, such as alcohol or nicotine. According to the World Health Organization, "There is no evidence whatsoever that caffeine has even remotely comparable physical and social consequences as those associated with serious drugs of abuse."

Cold Turkey!

Although moderate amounts of caffeine will not cause gastrointesintal ulcers to develop, if you already suffer from ulcers, caffeine may exacerbate these conditions by producing excess stomach acid. Talk to your doctor if you have any questions about how coffee might be affecting your health.

So you're drinking 1,250 mg a day? The biggest obstacle in your path is the withdrawal symptoms that often occur when you cut down the amount of caffeine you consume on a daily basis, an amount your body has come to expect. When your body doesn't get what it needs to start its engine, the following caffeine withdrawal symptoms may occur:

➤ headache

➤ drowsiness

➤ fatigue

➤ irritability

➤ depression

➤ nausea

➤ flu-like symptoms

The best way to avoid experiencing these symptoms is to slowly cut back on your caffeine consumption, using less and less every day. The following tips will help you get started:

➤ **Keep track.** Don't stop using your Daily Habit Log now! Even after you find out how much you're drinking, you'll need it to help you monitor when and why you pick up a cup, when and what symptoms occur.

➤ **Check labels.** You may be consuming far more caffeine than you realize. Make sure you know how much caffeine is in the food you eat, the beverages you drink, and the medication you take. The charts we provided earlier in this chapter will help, but learn to read labels and ask questions.

➤ **Take your time.** Doctors suggest that if you'd like to reduce the amount of caffeine you drink or eliminate it from your diet altogether, it's best to do so slowly, and spread it out over time by reducing the amount you consume 20 percent each week. (If you drink five cups of coffee a day, for instance, cut back just one cup a day the first week, another cup the next week, until you start to feel better.)

➤ **Switch to decaf (or lower-caf) beverages gradually.** If you're a coffee drinker, you can progressively switch from regular to decaf by mixing them before brewing. Mix in a higher proportion of decaf every day. Or switch to tea, which has less caffeine than coffee.

➤ **Less is more.** Drink your caffeine from smaller cups so you don't feel deprived even though you're drinking less.

➤ **Find healthy substitutes.** Postum or Pero are grain-based instant beverages that provide the richness and warmth of coffee, but without the caffeine. It may take awhile to get used to the difference, but when you adapt, you'll be pleased.

➤ **Avoid temptation.** Meeting friends for coffee at Starbucks probably isn't a good idea when you're trying to break your caffeine habit. Neither is looking at your trusty old Mr. Coffee sitting dormant on your kitchen counter every morning. Exploring new social alternatives and creating a caffeine-free home environment will help you stay on track.

➤ **Water, water everywhere.** Water is one of the most underrated health foods in the world—the noncaffeinated kind, anyway—and we urge you to drink as much as you can. Water helps flush out body toxins and hydrates your skin and other tissues.

➤ **Take a break.** To cope with the dips in energy you may feel as you taper your caffeine consumption, try taking a brisk walk outside or performing some easy stretches to get your blood flowing. Deep breathing exercises send oxygen to the blood and brain. If you're really sleepy and can manage it, take a nap, another highly underrated healthful activity.

The Zen of a Stress-Free Body and Mind

Short of a pilgrimage to Dharamsala in India to commune with the Dalai Lama, how can you achieve the Zen of a stress-free life? When you cut back on caffeine, you're on your way. As you turn to building alternative sources of energy, you'll find yourself moving around more, achieving a higher fitness level. Suddenly, you may find you're not clenching your jaw as tightly and your eyes aren't always popping out of your head. Maybe your stomach is more settled and you can concentrate on something for more than five minutes before getting irritated.

Sure, we'd all love a "magic pill" that gives us peace of mind and boundless energy at the same time. But, to date, humankind just hasn't found it. In the meantime, it's back to the basics of moderation and healthy living to reduce stress and promote productivity.

You may be surprised at how stimulating controlling caffeine can be!

The Least You Need to Know

➤ Caffeine is a powerful drug, with both risks and benefits.

➤ Many products besides coffee contain caffeine.

➤ Caffeine can make you feel more stressed-out instead of less stressed-out—when you need to relax the most!

➤ Slowly but surely cutting back on caffeine is the best way to reduce the amount you ingest, or to eliminate it from your diet altogether.

➤ There are plenty of healthy alternatives that generate the same productivity boost you get from caffeine.

133

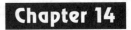

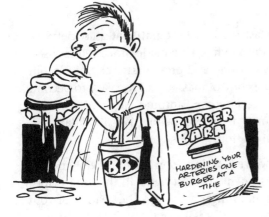

Food, Not So Glorious Food

Food. Weight. Body image. Too heavy. Too thin. We're never satisfied. Hey, could you pass me the ice cream?

It's ironic that in this land of plenty, at a time in history when, for most Americans, obtaining food is not a problem, food itself has become such an undermining force. Some people eat too much and for the wrong reasons; they gain weight, which threatens their health and their self-esteem. Other people avoid food, frightened, fearful, and in a state of self-denial. And a lot of people just eat whatever's convenient—without considering either nutritional value or taste.

How are *your* eating habits? Do you eat when you're hungry, or is your appetite triggered by other factors, such as anxiety, stress, or boredom? Do you enjoy what you eat, or do you feel angry, depressed, or fearful about food? Is exercise a regular part of your life, or does the food you eat immediately turn to fat instead of energy? Do you feel you've got a handle on proper nutrition, or could you use some help?

You Gotta Eat, Don't You?

It's not easy to have healthy food habits in our fast-food, instant gratification society. Advertising combined with the pressures of modern living have made processed foods— most of which are loaded with fat, sugar, empty calories, and preservative chemicals, our diet staples. America's love affair with the remote control makes it all too easy to become a couch potato junk-food junkie. Not to mention computers, automobiles, and auto- mated appliances, which keep us in our chairs more than ever before. We sit all day and we snack while we're doing it—not a good combination.

Because of all of these messages and obstacles, we've lost sight of what food really is and what it means to our health. First, food is nourishment. The nutrients in the food you eat every day are the catalysts for millions of major and minor miracles—the beating of your heart, the birth of an idea, the appreciation of taste and smell—that take place within your body.

Food is also a source of pleasure. We don't eat merely to ingest the various vitamins, minerals, and other substances we need to survive. Instead, eating is—and should be—a supremely sensual activity: We smell food's aromas, admire its colors and textures, taste its flavors, and feel its consistency inside our mouths. Meal times can also refresh our minds through conversation with family or tablemates. But too often these days, we're eating on the run, with little attention to how—or with whom—we're doing it.

The ABC's of Nutrition

Okay. Here's the bottom line about what you *need* to eat to stay healthy. The human body requires about 40 different essential nutrients to carry out its functions and main- tain its health. We also need about 2,000 calories a day (less if you're trying to lose weight or more if you're very active). Let's take a look at what they are:

> **Oxygen:** Surprise! Most of us take oxygen for granted, but study after study proves that the more oxygen you supply to your body's cells and to your brain—by breath- ing deeply and circulating more oxygen-rich blood during exercise—the better. (We'll talk more about exercise later.)
>
> **Daily requirement of oxygen:** As much as possible, naturally.
>
> **Water:** Water is found in almost everything we eat and drink; water regulates temperature, circulation, excretion, and aids in digestion. It bathes virtually all of our cells in moisture. Water also aids in the healthy process of weight loss by filling you up and helps to flush toxins out of your system.
>
> **Daily requirement of water:** 64 ounces (eight glasses).

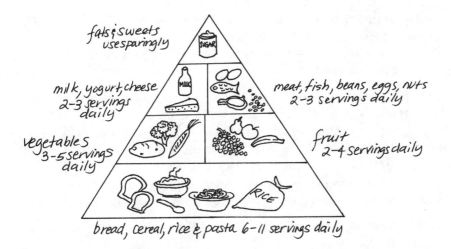

The Food Pyramid: A Healthy Eating Guide

Carbohydrates: Carbohydrates form the base of the USDA's Food Pyramid and should make up the bulk of a nutritious diet. Cereal, rice, pasta, bread, and whole grains are carbohydrates, as are fruits and vegetables (although the Food Pyramid puts fruits and vegetables into separate categories). Carbohydrates are the body's major source of energy. Dietary fiber is a type of carbohydrate that aids in digestion and helps keep the digestive tract clean and clear.

Daily Requirement of carbohydrates: 6–11 servings per day, (1 serving = 1 piece of bread or ½ cup of pasta or rice) or between 50 and 60 percent of your daily calories.

Fruits and vegetables: Fruits and vegetables are, with a few exceptions, low in fat and calories, high in fiber, and chock full of vitamins and minerals. They also can satisfy a craving for sweets (most fruits and certain vegetables) or carbohydrates (potatoes, yams, etc.).

Daily requirement of fruits and vegetables: 6 servings a day (1 serving = 1 small fruit or ½ cup cooked vegetables).

One Day at a Time
Fresh fruits and vegetables provide about 92 percent of the vitamin C and half the vitamin A in the nation's food supply, while contributing just 9 percent of the calories!

Protein: The term protein comes from the Greek word *protos*, which means first and foremost. Proteins are found in every body cell, constitute the most plentiful substance in the body of a normal-weight person, and make up about one-fifth of a normal adult's body weight. Meat, egg white, milk, and other animal products are rich in dietary protein, as are grains, and legumes (certain beans and peas, as well as tofu, made from soybeans).

Daily requirement of protein: 2–3 servings daily or 4 to 6 ounces total (25 percent of calories). Concentrate on lean protein (chicken, turkey, fish, lentils, dried peas, sprouts, grains, and egg whites) while avoiding whole eggs, red meat, and nuts, which are high in fat and cholesterol.

Dairy: Milk, yogurt, and cheese are our primary sources of an essential element, calcium. Calcium is necessary for proper blood clotting, helps to maintain blood pressure by controlling the contraction of blood vessel walls, and is essential to the health of bones, teeth, and nails. Most people neglect this part of their diet because dairy products also tend to be rather high in fat and calories. Fortunately, there are skim versions of these products that avoid this drawback. In addition, sardines and green leafy vegetables (kale, collard greens, broccoli, etc.) are also high in calcium.

Daily dairy requirement: 2–3 servings daily, at least 1,000 milligrams of calcium per day from non-dairy sources.

Fat: Get ready. Here's the only amount of fat you need in your diet to stay healthy: the equivalent of one tablespoon of olive oil a day. We're not kidding. That's all. This small amount performs important functions in the body, such as storing energy and carrying fat-soluble vitamins through the bloodstream. But most Americans have far too much fat in their diets. Research studies show that this gross amount of excess fat in the human diet is linked to breast cancer, colon cancer, heart disease—should we go on?

Daily requirements for fat: 9 grams a day. The American Heart Association and the USDA recommend that fat calories comprise no more than 20 percent of your total daily diet.

Notice what's missing altogether from our categories of essential nutrients? Sugar! Sugar has no nutritional value whatsoever. Plus, sugar sometimes converts to fat in the body. So, if you're eating a low-fat, high-sugar diet, you're kidding yourself. Want something sweet? Try a piece of fresh fruit instead.

When the Refrigerator Wins

So now you know what makes up a healthy diet and how you should portion your food on a daily basis. But that's not how it usually goes, is it? Maybe you give in to cravings, or find you overeat and gain weight, or maybe you shy away from eating out of fear, anxiety, or need for control.

When You Just Gotta Have It

Chocolate cake at midnight. Potato chips during the football game. That second (or third) serving of pasta. Food cravings can attack at any time.

A New Angle

A survey of college students at McMaster University in Hamilton Ontario found that 97 percent of the women and 68 percent of the men reported an occasional overwhelming desire for certain foods. Women are chocolate, bread, and ice cream lovers. Men go for red meat, potatoes, and pizza.

Food cravings have puzzled scientists for years. Recent research targets a complex combination of physical and emotional factors. For instance, our love of fat and fatty foods may well have evolved as a survival tactic: Throughout most of human history, people were hunters and gatherers who spent their time roaming around looking for food, and at the mercy of the elements. When they found fatty foods, they ate it, storing the excess to get them through the lean times. In today's society, however, food is *never* scarce, particularly fatty snack foods like cakes and cookies, and so, while natural, our craving for fat no longer serves a healthy purpose. Chemically speaking, foods are powerful substances that can change brain and body activity. Carbohydrates, such as potatoes, pasta, and grains, for example, are known to trigger the release of a brain chemical called serotonin. Serotonin elevates mood; in fact, many drugs used to treat depression act by boosting serotonin levels just like a bowl of pasta might. That may be why so many people tend to overeat when they're feeling depressed.

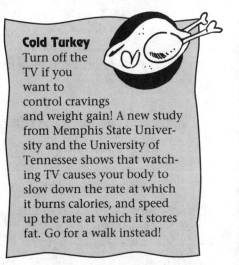

Cold Turkey
Turn off the TV if you want to control cravings and weight gain! A new study from Memphis State University and the University of Tennessee shows that watching TV causes your body to slow down the rate at which it burns calories, and speed up the rate at which it stores fat. Go for a walk instead!

But the power of suggestion is at work as well. Just hearing the theme music to a favorite TV show makes you want to break out the double chocolate chip ice cream. The sight of your boss's comments on your report triggers a craving for pizza so strong you spend the next hour imagining how it will taste when you get it home that night.

Fortunately, there're ways to manage food cravings so they don't get out of hand. Here are a few tips to get you started:

➤ **Acknowledge your cravings.** Everyone has food cravings, and everyone indulges them at one time or another. Denying that you have a desire for chocolate or pretzels or caviar is futile! Instead, indulge them in a moderate way: Have a single scoop of ice cream, two cookies, a handful of pretzels, a dollop of caviar.

➤ **Wait it out.** Cravings come and go—even if you don't indulge. Wait at least 10 minutes after your first twinges, and if you still want the food then, have half or less of the serving you crave.

➤ **Don't go hungry.** Eating on a regular basis—three larger or five smaller meals a day—will prevent many food cravings by keeping your stomach and brain satisfied.

➤ **Get moving.** Exercise relieves stress and distracts you from cravings. Take a walk, go out dancing, clean the bathroom with vigor!

➤ **Carry healthy snacks with you.** Eat an apple, peel a banana, or spoon up some fat-free yogurt.

➤ **Separate food from feelings, especially failure.** Remember the line from the movie *The Goodbye Girl*, "Starve a cold, feed a failure"? Instead of feeling our happiness or our depression, we eat instead. If eating to channel strong emotions is your modus operandi, make a pact to stay out of the kitchen when you're joyous, sad, angry, or frustrated and see what happens. Keep track of your reactions in your Daily Habit Log.

When You're Starving

It may be true that you can't be too rich, but being too thin, or wanting to be too thin, poses a significant hazard to your psychological and physical health. Many people—most of them women, although that is changing—avoid eating even the minimum daily requirement of nutrients in an effort to pare their body down to look like the impossible ideal of the 6-foot, 120-pound runway model.

Strictly Speaking
Anorexia nervosa is a psychological disorder characterized by an inability to, or strong aversion, toward food and eating. **Bulimia** is an eating disorder characterized by periods of binge eating, usually followed by purging by vomiting or use of laxatives or by periods of anorexia.

An urgent need to deny yourself food, or the enjoyment of food, can be dangerous to your physical and your mental health, causing eating disorders such as *anorexia nervosa* or *bulimia*. Take it easy on yourself, and try to accept the shape of your body the way it is naturally. We know that's easier said than done in a society that values thinness almost above all other physical attributes—even the late Princess Diana suffered from bulimia—but it's important to at least move toward a celebration of a healthy strong body. By doing so, you'll allow yourself to derive pleasure from eating once again.

When Too Much Is Never Enough

Today, more than 33 percent of Americans are obese (commonly defined as being 20 percent or more over their ideal body weight), a full 8 percent more than were obese just 15 years ago.

The health problems related to weight are myriad. Every pound over your ideal weight carries a greater risk for heart disease, hypertension, diabetes, and certain types of cancer.

A New Angle

Four recent Federal surveys of health practices indicate that 33 to 40 percent of adult women and 20 to 24 percent of men are currently trying to lose weight. Among men and women trying to lose weight, the reported time on a weight loss regimen in the past year averaged 6.4 and 5.8 months respectively, and the number of attempts to lose weight in the past two years averaged 2.5 and 2.0 attempts.

What about you? Is your eating going out of control? Take this quiz and see.

Are You a Compulsive Eater?

1. My life would be better if I could only lose weight.   *True*____   *False*____

2. I view food as comfort when I'm anxious, lonely, or angry.
   *True*____   *False*____

3. I keep eating even when I'm full.   *True*____   *False*____

4. If I ate whatever and whenever I wanted, I would be fat.
   *True*____   *False*____

5. My wardrobe consists only of clothes that hide as much of my body as possible.
   *True*____   *False*____

6. I often feel guilty after I eat.   *True* ____   *False*____

7. There're many foods I can't eat even a bite of because I'll lose control.
   *True*____   *False*____

8. I have tried many diets.   *True*____   *False*____

9. I think about food all the time.   *True*____   *False*____

10. I'm embarrassed about my enjoyment of food.   *True*____   *False*____

The more statements that ring true for you, the more likely it is that you're eating for the wrong reasons, and maybe gaining weight because of it.

Reality Log: You Are What You Eat

In a recent nutrition survey, 70 percent of people questioned said they had healthy diets. But when asked what they actually ate, researchers discovered that their diets were anything *but* healthy. What do *you* eat every day? When do you eat? Where? What do you think about and how do you feel while you're eating. That's right: back to the Daily Habit Log. Write it all down, every day for a week.

=My Daily Eating Log=

Monday

Time: 7:00 am
Food: Banana, cereal, skim milk
Feelings: Great! Revved me up
  and didn't weigh me down.

Time: 10:00 am
Food: Two donuts, two cups of
  coffee
Feelings: Needed an energy boost.
  Felt guilty but entitled.
  Got a headache later.

Time: Noon
Food: Small salad without dressing
Feelings: Doing penance for the
  sugar, fat & caffeine.
  Felt deprived and unsatisfied.

The Last 10 (or 30) Pounds

Without question, losing weight and keeping it off is one of the hardest tasks in the world. Only quitting smoking comes even close. If you're like most people with a weight problem in this country, for years you've tried and failed and tried and failed to lose those 10, 20, 30 or more pounds.

And what have you learned from all that hard work and disappointment? That diets don't work. You can eat only bananas or cabbage soup for three weeks, and maybe drop some pounds quickly, but pretty soon, your thighs or waistline expand once again.

The best way to eat well and maintain a healthy weight—or to lose weight if necessary—is to eat relatively small portions of a wide variety of foods and to exercise. That's it. Simple as that. Eat what you want (but not necessarily as *much* as you want) and get twenty to thirty minutes of cardiovascular exercise each day—even if that just means walking or marching in place. Sounds simple, doesn't it? But a lot of us are looking for a quicker solution that involves less effort and dedication. The most important tip of all is to make these changes a natural part of your life, so that the changes to your body come slowly but surely and last forever.

The Fat-Free Trap

It sounds too good to be true, and it is. First of all, most fat-free products are nutritionally empty anyway: Cookies, cakes, ice creams don't provide you with any essential nutrients and should be consumed in small amounts. And second—are you sitting down?—fat free doesn't mean you can eat a whole bag or box without getting fat! It doesn't mean that it's okay to eat four boxes of fat-free cookies instead of one box of "regular" cookies. If quantity is what you want, consider this: One cheeseburger's got as much fat as 50 apples, 30 cups of whole wheat pasta, or 80 cups of broccoli! So if you're eating the right kinds of nutritious, low-fat foods, you can eat more than just one and feel great.

Pills and Supplements

There just isn't a magic weight loss pill. There isn't one single dietary supplement or diet pill we'd recommend; we don't know a reputable doctor who would either. Sure, existing on a liquid diet for six months will allow you to drop some weight, but only on a temporary basis, since what's the first thing you'll do when you finish the diet? Eat, that's what. Eat and eat and eat some more, putting back on the pounds you lost and then some. Instead of asking your primary care physician for a diet pill or supplement, ask to be referred to a licensed nutritionist and work with your health care team to come up with a nutrition and exercise plan that makes sense for your health and fitness level. Then stick to it!

"You Mean I Have to Exercise????"

Yes. There's absolutely no way around it. If you don't, your body won't use the food-fuel you feed it in an efficient manner. Fitness icon Jack LaLanne put it this way: "You wouldn't use trash to fuel your car's engine. Why use the equivalent of nutritional trash to fuel your most precious earthly possession—your body!"

Exercise and Your Body

Exercise increases your overall fitness level, gives you more (not less!) energy, pumps more oxygen to the brain to help you think better and, believe it or not, feels good once you're used to it. Exercise also burns calories. The more you exercise, the more you can eat. In fact, obese people actually eat an average of 600 calories *less* every day than active people of normal weight. If that isn't enough to get you going, then we don't know what is!

What Kind of Shape Are You In?

Take this short quiz to see just how fit you are today:

1. When you sprint up a flight of stairs are you:

    (a) Seeing stars, and we don't mean Arnold Schwarzenegger or Jane Fonda.

    (b) Ready and able to carry on a conversation.

    (c) Prepared to tackle at least another flight.

2. If you sit on the floor with your legs straight in front of you and your toes pointing toward the ceiling, are you able to:

    (a) Touch your knees, but only if you really try.

    (b) Touch your calves.

    (c) Reach past your feet.

3. How many push-ups can you do?

    (a) I can't get down on the floor in the first place.

    (b) Ten, but only the "girl" kind.

    (c) Ten one-arms, like Jack Palance at the Oscars.

4. Moving as quickly as you can, how fast can you walk a mile?

    (a) Do you think it's a mile to my front door?

    (b) About 20 minutes.

    (c) Fifteen minutes or less.

5. How many minutes a day do you perform activities that cause your heart rate to rise and perspiration to occur?

    (a) Does watching an exciting episode of my soap opera count?

    (b) About 15 minutes.

    (c) More than 30 minutes.

How did you do? Remember, consult your physician before beginning any exercise regimen. If you scored mostly:

A's   You've got a long way to go. You've been a couch potato for some time, and your heart, lungs, and muscles need some love and attention.

B's   Exercise isn't foreign to you. You've been there and done that, but so far your heart's not really in it. Start increasing the number of times you exercise each week (aim for at least three or four times) and the amount of time you spend at each session (at least 30 to 45 minutes).

C's   You're really on your way. Keep it up.

Working Out

It's not so hard to make exercise a part of your life. Try these strategies to get you started:

➤ **Fit it in, gently.** Exercise isn't an all-or-nothing proposition. You don't have to run every single morning, or make every evening's aerobics class. Your daily exercise can consist of a brisk walk to the market, an afternoon of gardening, even an hour of vigorous housecleaning—any activity that requires your body to move and your heart rate to rise.

➤ **Schedule time to exercise.** For many people, exercise is often last on a long list of "things to do" and thus the first to go when things get busy. Consider exercise sessions like business appointments you've made with yourself—and keep them.

➤ **Accent the positive.** Perhaps the most important element in the design of any long-term fitness plan is choosing activities you enjoy and that leave you feeling refreshed and motivated. Experiment with a few different sports, exercise classes, and activities until you find one or more that inspire you to keep at it.

➤ **Remember that exercise lifts depression.** Exercising releases substances into your body that elevate your mood. As yoga guru Joan Budilovsky, author of *The Complete Idiot's Guide to Yoga*, says, "Feeling great: meditate. Feeling down: Move around!"

The Refrigerator, Unchained

Balance. Structure. Satisfaction. When all is said and done, these three principles are the heart of a healthy diet and a healthy relationship to food. Think about the following points and then make an appointment to discuss a diet and exercise program with your doctor.

Balance

➤ **Follow the guidelines of the USDA's Food Pyramid.**

➤ **Maintain a healthy weight.** By gaining control over your food cravings, learning to enjoy instead of fear food, and by adding exercise to your life, you'll soon be able to better manage your weight.

➤ **Consume all good things in moderation.** Unless you've got a specific allergy or sensitivity, no food is off-limits—as long as you practice portion control.

Structure

➤ **Set regular times for your meals.** Whether you choose to eat three moderate-sized meals or five smaller meals per day, give yourself time to sit down and really enjoy the food you eat rather than just grab something.

➤ **Plan and cook ahead.** Time has a way of flying by. If you make the effort to plan ahead by creating a menu, shopping, and even cooking ahead of time, you'll stand a better chance of resisting the temptation to pick up whatever food is at hand, regardless of its nutritional value or even its appeal to your taste buds.

➤ **Plan special meals and treats.** Although we should all aim to eat healthy, wholesome foods as often as possible, many of us have cravings for foods that are less than ideal. Never completely deprive yourself of the foods you crave, but instead build in some occasional indulgences into your diet.

Satisfaction

➤ **Add variety to your diet.** By eating lots of different kinds of food during the day, you'll not only improve your chances of getting all the nutrients you need, you'll probably find yourself enjoying your diet more than ever before. At least once a week, try a new food—an exotic fruit or vegetable, for example—or cook a different dish.

➤ **Take the time to enjoy the sensual aspects of eating.** Eating food on the run means denying yourself the pleasure of setting an elegant table and lingering over a fine meal in the company of family and friends. At least once in awhile, take the time to make eating an experience to be savored rather than an automatic activity.

➤ **Eat foods that leave you feeling healthy and well.** Nutritious food, prepared well and eaten in a relaxed atmosphere nourishes your body and your soul.

The Least You Need to Know

➤ Eating well is a complicated activity in today's society.

➤ Keeping track of your eating habits will help you gain control over your diet.

➤ Fat and sugar are a dangerous duo that can add pounds without optimum nutritional benefit.

➤ Thirty minutes of activity every day—from taking a walk to working out at the gym—helps you lose pounds and keep them off.

➤ Establishing balance, maintaining structure, and striving for satisfaction should be your dietary goals.

Part 4
Stop Driving Me (and Everyone Else) Crazy!

Has telling those little white lies become second nature to you? Have you ever met an appointment you weren't late for? Do you find that your relationships with family members, friends, and romantic companions are fraught with problematic interactions?

If a lack of communication and organizational skills prevents you from meeting your personal and professional goals, there are some simple (though not necessarily easy!) techniques you can use to break those bad habit tendencies, establish some better skills, and head toward a more successful future.

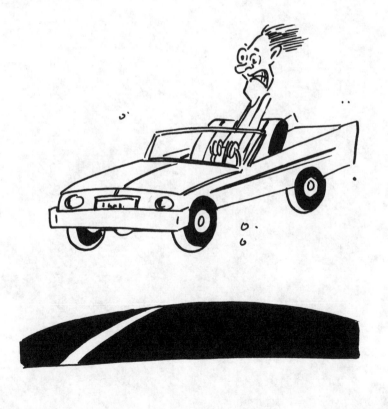

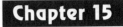

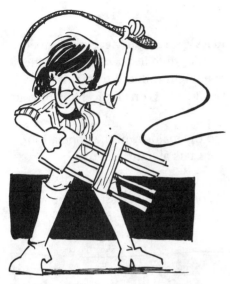

Chapter 15

Tame Those Tendencies

In This Chapter

➤ Admitting to your inclinations

➤ Identifying your negative patterns

➤ How your tendencies affect your relationships

➤ Taking responsibility

The word "tendency" sounds innocent enough. The dictionary's definition seems benign: "An inclination to act or think in a particular way." What's wrong with that? Well, potentially, nothing. And, potentially, everything. Back in Chapter 3, "But I Like It Like That," we talked about tendencies as a way of displacing frustration or anxiety, and those are the kind of tendencies that can become bad habits. You don't have to worry about your tendency to say "please" or your tendency to prefer a steamed vegetable platter to a double bacon cheeseburger. But your tendency to throw a dish against the wall every time your sister makes you feel academically inferior or your tendency to start your research for that 30-page term paper the night before it's due are different matters altogether.

"Me? I Don't Have Tendencies..."

Maybe you think you don't have any negative tendencies. "Sure, I can never remember important dates and I firmly believe in the power of a little white lie every now and then, but I don't have any bad tendencies people notice," you might think. What's this? Do we detect a little hesitation as you not-quite-confidently assure us no one notices any of your bad habits?

Well, maybe you're right. Maybe you appear faultless to the majority of the population. But let's take a different approach, just for a minute. Let's talk about your goals.

What do you want in life? Who do you plan to become? Where do you want to be next year? In 5 years? In 10 years? And are you on your way, or are you, at least to some extent, spinning your wheels?

A New Angle

Maslow's **hierarchy of motivation** ranked human drives that must be fulfilled, usually in order (although the hierarchy is dynamic), before humans can reach their full potential.

1. Physiological: Hunger, thirst, shelter, etc.

2. Safety: Feeling secure and protected from harm.

3. Social: Affection, acceptance, etc.

4. Esteem: Also called ego, esteem involves self-respect, achievement, recognition, status, etc.

5. Self-actualization: Achieving one's creative human potential.

Abraham Maslow, a psychologist famous for developing a *hierarchy of motivation*, studied the lives of highly effective people, noticing that "What a man can be, he must be." Since he said this in the 1950s, we'll forgive his sexist language and move on to examine his view: He and his colleague, Carl Rogers broke with their predecessors in psychology who believed that all human actions are ruled by the unconscious, by primitive urges (these were Sigmund Freud's ideas), or by the environment. Maslow, on the other hand, believed that humans are masters of their own destinies, and that every human has the potential for, and indeed ultimately is motivated by, the desire for self-actualization. Maslow believed we can make independent, proactive choices that will shape our destinies, and that after our basic, primary needs are met, self-actualization is the ultimate human goal.

What does this have to do with tendencies, you might ask? Everything! All bad habits hold you back from being your best, but negative behavioral tendencies do more than eat up your time or your financial resources. They compromise your relationships and even your integrity. Denying them is a way of avoiding responsibility for who you are and your potential for success and progress. Maintaining them is like erecting stumbling blocks in the center of your path toward self-actualization. After all, how can you achieve your human potential if you can't even get to work on time?

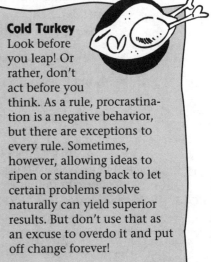

Cold Turkey
Look before you leap! Or rather, don't act before you think. As a rule, procrastination is a negative behavior, but there are exceptions to every rule. Sometimes, however, allowing ideas to ripen or standing back to let certain problems resolve naturally can yield superior results. But don't use that as an excuse to overdo it and put off change forever!

Maybe you put off those household chores until the bathtub sports more mildew than porcelain, or you blow off steam by snapping at your spouse about minor inconveniences, or you periodically forget your son's baseball game, or you've just told your boss you missed your deadline because of a "family emergency" again. Whatever your negative tendencies, they're distracting you from achieving your goals and undermining your self-esteem and sense of integrity. If you seek them out and jettison them, you can get on to the bigger business of really living!

When the Rest of the World Has the Real Problem

"No, no," you say, "I really don't do any of those things—at least not when I can help it." Unfortunately, your tendency to shift the blame away from yourself may just be another bad habit! Sure, you take credit for your triumphs and assume responsibility for your actions when things are going well—and you should—but it's all too easy to pass the buck when life is less than sunny.

Let's face it: Your life is your own. Have you ever said, or even thought, anything similar to the following statements?

➤ I could have finished this project if people hadn't been (calling me all night long, wanting my help on their own projects, asking me for favors, telling me what to do and how to do it).

➤ Society is too fast-paced and demanding for me. That's why I can't (stay organized, make it to work on time, keep my checkbook balanced, keep the kitchen clean, stay in touch with my friends).

➤ My boss has unrealistic expectations, so of course I can't (accomplish all the tasks in my job description, give a top-notch presentation, secure that account, finish that report, get that promotion).

➤ I only get angry like that when I'm provoked.

➤ I would never have to lie if (society didn't have such unreasonable rules, my spouse truly understood me, my job had a more flexible environment, my parents weren't so strict, my friends weren't so moralistic).

See how easy it is to transfer blame? It's no wonder that it becomes such a nasty habit. But taking responsibility for yourself means admitting your mistakes and recognizing your shortcomings as well as reaping the kudos. Next time you find yourself blaming someone or something else for anything—anything at all—stop and ask yourself if you just might be responsible for the situation. Then consider the consequences of owning up. Would it really be so bad? Couldn't the benefits outweigh the risks? You might earn a little more respect—and a little self-respect, too—from the people you deal with than you've received so far. And the discomfort you feel fessing up might stick with you, so passing the buck won't be as easy the next time. Lying, making excuses, denying, putting off, and blowing up may not seem like appropriate responses for much longer!

A New Angle

According to a *USA Today* poll, nearly 90 percent of adults say it is hard for them to tell a lie, although 24 percent say lying is sometimes justified. How often do people say they lie?

➤ Hardly ever: 68 percent

➤ Occasionally: 17 percent

➤ Never: 11 percent

➤ Frequently: 3 percent

The question is, were they lying to the pollsters?

Looking Inward: A Self-Test Challenge

Tendencies cover a wide range of behavioral phenomena, although most can be grouped into just two categories: The absence of effective communication, and that ubiquitous tendency to procrastinate. Take the following self-test to uncover your own particular proclivities.

1. You've just given a stunningly successful dinner party, but the dishes are piled to the ceiling. After the last guest departs, you survey the mess, and:

   (a) Feel extremely irritated. The least your guests could have done after that wonderful dinner you provided would be to rinse off their own plates. No one even offered to pitch in and help clean up! What rude and ungrateful friends you have.

   (b) Take one brief look at the mess, then turn away in despair and go to bed. Concentrate on how great the party was. You'll deal with the mess later.

   (c) Tell your spouse or roommate that if only they would've rinsed the dishes as people stacked them in the kitchen, you wouldn't have this mess to contend with.

   (d) Tell your spouse or roommate you have a killer headache, and coerce him or her into cleaning the mess up for you while you go off to sleep. Sure, you'll feel a little guilty.

2. You've just been assigned a huge research project, due in six weeks. As your boss or teacher maps out the assignment, deep down you know that you'll:

   (a) Think of ideas for exactly five weeks and five days, then spend a sleepless weekend cramming together the bare minimum. Who knows—maybe your genius lies in being under pressure!

   (b) Probably be attending the funeral of an imaginary great aunt—to whom you were desperately attached—in just about six weeks' time.

   (c) Cough up 50 bucks and give it to your best friend—an expert at research—to do the legwork, and maybe even some of the writing. Heck, why not add a couple of bucks a page and have the thing typed, too?

   (d) Immediately begin to feel irritated that you have to take on a project this big. As if you have nothing else to do! Before the project has been completely explained, you're already fuming.

3. You told an acquaintance you couldn't get together with her tonight because you had to stay home and get some work done. She's just so tedious sometimes! Alas, you run into her in a restaurant, where you're dining with one of your more interesting friends. She sees you, and looks hurt. You:

   (a) Turn bright red, apologize profusely, and then whisper, out of your interesting friend's earshot, that he was in desperate need and you had no choice but to take him out to dinner to talk to him about his problem.

   (b) Even if you've met her eyes, you quickly look beyond her and pretend, with every ounce of your being, that you don't see her. Then leave ASAP, even if you've already ordered. You can always eat somewhere else.

   (c) Feel furious. How dare she be at the same restaurant! Give her the evil eye from across the room, letting her know she's obviously done something wrong. If she approaches you, you'll act disgusted and refuse to talk to her.

   (d) Dash up to her as if she's your long-lost best friend, and spew forth whatever excuses you can think of: that handy imaginary aunt just died and you're out making funeral arrangements, your companion is really your probation officer, or she absolutely must swear not to remember she saw you there because you're on a top secret mission for the CIA. Then, promise her you'll do lunch next week. (That gives you a week to think of a new excuse.)

4. Speaking of habits, your significant other is doing that thing again with his or her knuckles. You're trying to concentrate on a really good book, but that sound is about to drive you straight up the wall. You:

   (a) Get up and leave the room. You can read somewhere else.

   (b) Listen to the horrible sound for about 30 minutes, then explode with something like, "If you don't stop that disgusting sound immediately, I'm going to be sick all over the floor!" Or, alternatively, you get up and leave the room, but not before knocking over a book or two, and slamming the door so hard the walls shake.

   (c) Tell your significant other that you're feeling ill. Could he/she possibly run out and pick up some antacid? (Anything to get the source of that sound out of the house!)

   (d) Pretend to call your mother, then mention that your mother was wondering what that horrible sound was, and that she also said cracking your knuckles will give you arthritis. "Mother says it's in your best interest to stop, honey!"

5. Everything is piling up at once. Your boss is pushing for you to put in some over-time, your three kids all need to be driven somewhere at 3:30 p.m., the washing machine just started to make a strange grinding sound, and the car battery is dead. Now you think you hear the dog throwing up in the vicinity of your brand new living room carpet. You are most likely to react by:

   (a) Calling in sick for work (you can fake a really convincing cough), telling your family your boss needs you for the day (instructing them not to bother you at work under any circumstances), then taking off for a long drive in the country. And then ending the day with a leisurely stop at the mall. After all, you need a break, and no one would understand the truth, anyway.

   (b) Telling your boss that your child is sick so you can't put in overtime, convincing a couple of friends with station wagons or mini-vans to play chauffeur to your kids because they owe you, suggesting your significant other do a load of laundry ("I didn't hear any strange noise, honey,") and asking your oldest child to go check on Rover (he who finds a mess courtesy of the dog has to clean it up). Hey, today doesn't seem so stressful after all!

   (c) Convincing yourself that you can get that extra work done later, you've got enough clean clothes to last for another few days, and what're buses for, anyway, if not for transportation! And maybe if you don't go look in the living room, whatever's there will just...go away?

   (d) Blowing up, screaming at your kids, booting the dog outside, venting your rage at your local appliance repair technician and at the mechanic who comes to jump-start your car, and then, in a final and satisfying finale, smashing something really expensive into an infinite number of tiny shards.

Circle your answers, then determine which column has the most circles. Then read on to discover your tendency profile.

Tendency Scorecard

Question	There's Always Tomorrow	Blowin' Off Steam	Pants on Fire!	Passin' the Buck
1.	B	A	D	C
2.	A	D	B	C
3.	B	C	D	A
4.	A	B	C	D
5.	C	D	A	B

There's Always Tomorrow. You're a master procrastinator. You put off unpleasant chores and situations as long as possible, and sometimes even deny they exist, when you can. Even if you've become accomplished at doing an adequate job at the last minute, or averting certain situations by ignoring them, you aren't living up to your potential. Whether you procrastinate because you're simply disorganized or because you've got a serious problem confronting certain issues, this is a habit to begin conquering TODAY! You won't believe how much more smoothly your life can run, and how much more you can put into projects, chores, and even relationships, if you work on them for awhile rather than rushing through under deadline or avoiding confrontations. Nothing is done well at the last minute, and no relationship can thrive on denial.

Blowin' Off Steam. Maybe you've got a little problem with your temper—but don't take it personally, and please don't throw this book across the room—we're only saying this to help you! Whether you tend to have full-blown tantrums or a simple, low-but-constant level of irritation, anger is a momentous obstacle to your happiness and success. You need an attitude adjustment, and you need it fast. But don't think it's as easy as merely *deciding* to change. Anger can have its roots in many things, and you may need some time to uncover the source of your negativity. Give it time, and be patient with yourself. Breathe! Relax. Practice stress management. You can work it out, and you're worth it. No one should have to feel angry and frustrated all the time.

Pants on Fire! All right, admit it: You tend to bend the truth now and then. Sometimes, you even snap it right in two. Of course, very occasional lying is excusable, especially if it's to spare someone's feelings and the lie truly doesn't hurt anyone—including your own sense of integrity. But re-creating truth has now become part of your daily routine, and you may well have a problem taking responsibility for your actions. Learning to be honest is a challenge, but living without lies will set you free. You'll never have to re-member what you told to whom, and you'll never have to scramble for believable fiction to remedy every uncomfortable situation. Instead, you'll learn to face the truth and move on. It's much simpler, and people will finally be able to trust you—and you'll be able to trust yourself.

Passin' the Buck. Avoiding problems and stress by passing them on to someone else is a cop-out and can become addictive. It's so easy to subtly suggest your sister was the one who forgot to book the rehearsal hall, or your secretary never gave you the phone mes-sage, or your child is sick so you'll just have to stay home. Passing the buck often goes hand in hand with lying. Both are ways to avoid truth and its inevitable consequences. Maybe you think passing blame to someone else is fine if that person won't suffer. After all, what boss is going to call your home and scream at your supposedly sick five-year-old? But refusing to take responsibility for your own actions compromises your integrity. Learning to face the consequences of your actions will bring you to a new level of matu-rity—not a boring, stodgy maturity, but an empowering maturity where you control your own life.

You Can't Change Your Relationships Until You Change Yourself

Now that you've got a better idea of what kind of negative behavioral tendencies you gravitate toward, we'd like you to expand your view of your habit beyond your own life and consider how it affects your relationships. All the previously mentioned bad habits affect relationships in profound ways, and recognizing this may be just the extra push you need to commit to change.

A concept we discussed in Chapter 1, "What Is a Bad Habit?" and in Chapter 2, "Why You Do the Things You Do," applies here as well: procrastinating, losing your temper, and shifting responsibility are all passive-aggressive behaviors. You're expressing anger, disappointment, and/or frustration with yourself, with your relationships, or with your life circumstances in inappropriate ways.

The procrastinator may procrastinate for any number of reasons, but the other people in a procrastinator's life will all suffer similarly—and that may be part of your motivation if you tend to put things off. If you fail to start (or complete) household responsibilities, wait until the last minute to complete projects, or embrace cramming as your primary study skill, the consequences don't just affect you. The people you live with will suffer from a household in chaos. The people you love will learn they can't depend on you to get things done. Your higher-ups—your bosses and/or teachers—will turn to more organized and dependable people, and guess who'll get the good recommendations and the juicy promotions? Not you.

One Day at a Time

Having trouble getting yourself to clean the house? Try a trick from a friend who is an admittedly compulsive cleaner, and assign one room to each day of the week. If you know you only have to tackle the bathroom or the bedroom today, the task may not seem as daunting. You can even assign a bigger chore for the first or last week of every month: January means cleaning out the hall closet, May means washing the outsides of all the windows, August means painting the porch, etc.

If you can't make yourself load the dishwasher or write up a simple report until the zero hour, how can anyone expect you to put consistent time and energy into a relationship? Chances are, they won't expect it, and if they do, you'll disappoint them again and again, even if only in the minor details of life. Ten years of "forgetting" to wipe food off the kitchen counter or call your mother can add up to a seriously damaged relationship. Could it be that you're really angry at your mother? Or crave another kind of relationship with her?

The angry person makes an equally difficult partner, parent, sibling, and child. People may learn to tiptoe around you to keep from inciting your wrath. They may hide what's really going on from you for their own protection. You can never have a fully developed relationship with someone who can't be open with you for fear of what you'll do. Controlling your anger isn't being dishonest. The "angry you" isn't the "real you," it's the you caught up in an intense emotion that prohibits you from more rational thinking. Letting your anger pass away without allowing it to hurt anyone (or destroy any more property!) is an important step toward learning how to interact on a deeper level with others.

Lying *compromises* relationships for obvious reasons. If you lie, people won't trust you, and if your loved ones can't trust you, you don't have a truly functional relationship with them. First and foremost, tackle lying to those who're most important to you. They deserve to know the truth about who you are, what you've done, what you haven't done, and what they mean to you. Honest relationships are strong relationships, and if honesty tears a relationship apart, chances are, it was weak to begin with. (There're a few exceptions—even "Dear Abby" advises against telling all truths, all the time. But in general, truth is best.)

Strictly Speaking
The word **compromise** has two very distinct definitions: You can compromise with a partner by agreeing to meet him or her halfway, or you can compromise a relationship or your own integrity by performing a negative, undermining action.

Shifting blame and responsibility onto others is evidence that you can't handle—or that you actually fear—the rigors of a serious relationship. If you can't admit you forgot that important meeting or that it was your turn to drive the carpool, how can you admit to those closest to you that you've been unreasonable or insensitive or just plain wrong? Admitting that you're wrong or that you've made a mistake isn't easy, but it's crucial for healthy relationships. If one person is always "right," the relationship will be one-sided and eventually disintegrate, or worse, maintain itself but with two miserable participants. Start taking responsibility for your actions with the ones you love. Soon, you'll learn to transfer this important skill—this new "habit"—to all aspects of your life.

Are you beginning to understand how your negative tendencies affect you and your relationships? In the chapters that follow, we'll examine the issues we've touched on in further depth. For now, the important thing is to recognize them, then tackle them. Do it for your friends, your family, your significant other—but most importantly, do it for yourself. Becoming the master of your own destiny isn't selfish. It's the best way to spend your time on this Earth!

The Least You Need to Know

➤ Negative tendencies such as procrastination, lying, or losing one's temper can become bad habits that undermine self-esteem and undercut relationships.

➤ It's easy to blame your behavior on other people or your environment, but accepting responsibility for your actions will make you a stronger and more trustworthy person.

➤ You can learn to minimize your negative tendencies, and by doing so, improve the quality of your relationships and attain your emotional and practical goals.

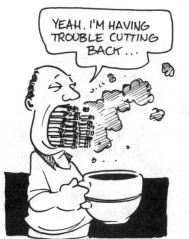

YEAH. I'M HAVING TROUBLE CUTTING BACK...

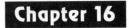

Chapter 16

Be Straightforward

In This Chapter

> ➤ Bad habits that undermine relationships

> ➤ Little white lies and big whoppers, forgetting about it, and losing your cool

> ➤ New strategies for better communication

We're gonna give it to you straight: It isn't always easy to be truthful with yourself or straightforward with others. The truth hurts, at least often enough to discourage us from automatically revealing our true feelings and motivations. Instead, some of us develop the bad habit of hiding them, either by lying, by conveniently "forgetting," or by expressing anger in order to distract ourselves and others from the reality of the situation. Does this describe you?

Fortunately, there's a solution: Face the truth and express it as often as possible. Easy? Not at all. Worth it? Absolutely. The truth *will* set you free. You'll no longer have to hide your genuine feelings or desires from your family, friends, and colleagues—or, for that matter, from yourself. Not a bad payoff for a little discomfort now and then! Let's find out how to go about it.

Little White Lies and Big Whoppers

First of all, don't beat yourself up too much if you've fallen into the habit of—well, there's no other way to put it—lying. The practice is virtually endemic in our society today. We've come to accept that politicians lie (and not just to save someone's feelings). Cheating on spouses, income taxes, and job applications is considered pretty run of the mill. Lying is the easiest way in the world to avoid unpleasant consequences of all kinds.

But without a doubt, the habit of saying something that's not true will eventually erode your relationships, as well as your own sense of self. It may be a cliché these days, but no healthy relationship of any kind can exist for long without honesty and trust.

Relationships can suffer from more than the obvious "Honey, I have to work late tonight" kind of lies. People lie—even to the people they love—for any number of reasons. When it comes to avoiding hurting someone's feelings (such as by saying a haircut looks great when you know it won't look fine for another week or two), "stretching the truth" might be okay. But if you lie in order to avoid conflict in your relationships or to protect yourself from natural repercussions, you're at the least taking the lazy way out and at worst deceiving yourself and the people in your life. You certainly won't be able to work out your relationship problems, and you'll be providing your loved ones and colleagues a false sense of who you are and what's important to you.

Miguel de Unamuno, a Spanish philosophical writer who lived around the turn of the century, once said, "To fall into a habit is to begin to cease to be." This is especially true of lying. Building a life on lies is like building that proverbial castle in the sand. It won't hold, and sooner or later, it's going to cave in.

There are many reasons to lie, and all kinds of situations in which lying comes in "handy." If lying is your bad habit, see if any of the following scenarios ring true.

Deceptions and Subterfuges

This type of lie is the most obvious one: It quite purposely hides the truth so you can gain an advantage or reach a goal. Have you ever lied to purposefully mislead someone?

➤ "I'm single." (When the picture of your spouse and toddler is burning a hole in your pocket as your hand slides over a companion's shoulders.)

➤ "I loved Yale—it was so academically and intellectually challenging." (When your chances of getting a job begin to wither and two years of community college simply won't do.)

➤ "I'll call you, I promise."(When you know your hand will fall off before you pick up the phone and dial that number.)

➤ "It's never been worn. I brought it home and it just didn't look right anymore." (While you're praying the salesperson doesn't spot the stain on the back of the jacket.)

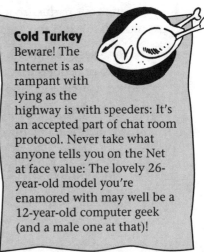

Cold Turkey
Beware! The Internet is as rampant with lying as the highway is with speeders: It's an accepted part of chat room protocol. Never take what anyone tells you on the Net at face value: The lovely 26-year-old model you're enamored with may well be a 12-year-old computer geek (and a male one at that)!

The Grand Gesture

Do you say things you don't mean to provoke a reaction from the person you're communicating with? See if you've flung any of these comments out during an exchange:

➤ "I hate you!" (To incite anger.)

➤ "I was the hit of the party. Too bad you didn't show up!" (To incite jealousy or remorse.)

➤ "You look like you've lost weight!" (To endear yourself to someone. Don't fool yourself: If the statement is untrue, and your friend didn't ask you about his weight, you're not saying it just to make him "feel good about himself.")

➤ "You're absolutely right and I'm wrong." (To facilitate the end of a fight.)

Make It Go Away

As you know by now, most bad habits develop out of the need to avoid—consequences, stress, anxiety, fear, disappointment, you name it. Have you ever lied in any of these situations?

➤ "These shoes only cost $25—it won't cut into our rent money!" (To avoid an argument, temporarily, until the bill comes.)

➤ "I swear I didn't see any stop sign, Officer!" (To avoid responsibility, even if she gives you a ticket anyway.)

➤ "I can do the job for $5,000." (To get out of a job you don't want to tackle—even though you know you could do it for $2,000—but don't want to argue with, or disappoint, a client.)

➤ "You are absolutely right and I'm wrong." (To avoid a fight in the first place.)

Catching Yourself in the Act

Lies come in many forms and trigger many different outcomes. If having an affair is your goal, then lying about your marital status gets you want you want—for awhile anyway.

Telling your partner that he's right and you're wrong will help avoid or avert an argument, but leaves the deeper issues still there to resolve in the future.

Nevertheless, like all "good" bad habits, lying allows you to avoid the immediate consequences or feelings that would otherwise emerge with the truth. In this way, it can be seductive, tempting, and indeed addictive.

Do you find it all too easy to lie? Has lying become a bad habit for you? Find out by answering the following questions:

1. Have you, on more than one occasion, prefaced a lie with, "You won't believe this in a million years, but I swear it's true!"?   Yes____   No____

2. Do you sometimes lie just because you think a lie would be more interesting than the truth?   Yes____   No____

3. Do you ever lie without intending to beforehand—it just slips right out? Yes____   No____

4. Do you ever start to believe your own lies?   Yes____   No____

5. Do you lie almost every day to avoid some kind of consequence? Yes____   No____

6. Do you ever get the feeling people don't believe what you're saying? Yes____   No____

7. Do you ever want to tell the truth about something, but find yourself unable to? Yes____   No____

If you've answered "yes" to three or more of the above questions, lying is a bad habit for you and your lies may be controlling your life. Now is the time to embrace truth as your new modus operandi.

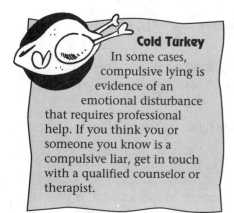

Cold Turkey
In some cases, compulsive lying is evidence of an emotional disturbance that requires professional help. If you think you or someone you know is a compulsive liar, get in touch with a qualified counselor or therapist.

Maybe you've discovered that you only tell a fib or two on occasion. Is it still wrong? That depends. Do you think you know the difference between a "white lie" and a "big whopper"? After each item in the following list, mark a WL if you think the statement is a "white lie" and perfectly excusable, and mark a BW if you think it's a lie that compromises either you or the person being lied to:

➤ "I left my report/presentation/term paper on the train!" (You haven't started it yet.)

➤ "Your baby is adorable!" (You think it must be a baby, but it sure looks a lot more like a possum!)

➤ "You never do anything nice for me!" (Just last week, he/she gave you a really nice back rub, and who did the dishes yesterday?)

➤ "I didn't see anything, Officer!" (You were driving by just as that car was rear-ended.)

➤ The grocery store clerk accidentally gives you an extra $10. (You notice, but walk quickly away.)

➤ You forget to make an important call to a client. (When you remember, you call with the excuse that you had to leave the office unexpectedly and missing the appointment was unfortunately unavoidable.)

> **Strictly Speaking**
> A **white lie** describes a lie about a trivial matter, often told to spare someone's feelings. Not all white lies are benign, however, because they can create false impressions and misconstrued relationships.

➤ You arrive very late to a dinner party and tell the hostess you were in a minor fender bender. (Everyone is okay, thank goodness!)

➤ You forget your best friend's birthday, so you dash off a note promising an un-named big surprise, and put it in an envelope. (She'll never know it wasn't planned all along, and you've bought yourself some time.)

No need to add up your score here because—except for the compliment about your friend's baby (which is pretty much required)—all the rest are unacceptable.

"No!" you protest. "I should be able to lie to keep my job, or at least to keep from hurting my hostess's or best friend's feelings!" We hate to burst your bubble, but these are classic examples of refusing to accept the consequences for your actions. Look at it this way: Telling the truth may make you feel extremely embarrassed and uncomfortable in the short term. Or it may require an investment of time and effort that you just don't want to make. But hey, don't you prefer it when people are honest with you? Don't you *expect* it? And—let's face it—when you know you have to come clean, you'll be far less likely to get yourself into a situation that requires a lie again.

Keeping Track of the Truth

We hope you're beginning to see that lots of lies most people deem "white" are really pretty big whoppers, at least cumulatively or in the long run. But we all know that forcing yourself to feel discomfort and embarrassment isn't exactly great incentive to stop lying. "I'll experience more pain? Sure, I'll stop!" you scoff. See, there's another lie!

No, we have a better strategy, assuming you really are committed to breaking your bad habit. Starting today, keep a Truth Log (we like to accentuate the positive, or else we'd call it a Lying Log). You can simply rename your Daily Habit Log from Chapter 5, "Step 1:

Identify the Behavior," or create a new notebook or computer file devoted to this exercise. At the end of the chapter, we provide you with an example of how your Daily Habit Log might look if communication problems like lying and losing your temper add up to your bad habit.

For one week, at the end of each day, write down everything you remember you said or did that wasn't completely honest. Don't worry about doing anything other than recording your "lying incidences" for one week. The point is to become aware of when you are lying, because chances are, you don't even realize it half the time.

After one week, go back and read over what you've written. Does it sound like you have a problem? On to Step 2! This week, continue to write down every untruth, then after it, write what you could have said that would've been honest. Don't worry about really doing it. Just write it down. This will get you thinking about creative solutions and also acquaint you with what the consequences of your actions would be if you took responsibility.

Step 3 is the tough one. By now, you'll probably be much more aware that you're about to lie before the words come out of your mouth. When you feel a lie coming on, think of a better way, then give it a try. Really try. Commit. And chances are, by now, you'll be less likely to get yourself into situations where lying is necessary, since you're now so accustomed to considering the consequences.

We know it sounds like a difficult process, but think of it this way: Three easy weeks to a more honest you!

Forgetting About It

So you forgot to take out the trash? You forgot to pay the bills? You forgot your anniversary? Maybe consciously you believe you actually do forget things a lot. "Give me a break—I'm absent-minded," you might wish to inform us. Guess what? We don't buy it. Absent-mindedness is a bad habit, and it's also a miscommunication with yourself that leads to the disappointment of others. You aren't obligated to forget. You aren't genetically predisposed to forget. Forgetting has quite simply become a convenient bad habit.

Assuming responsibility for even the most mundane (to you) details of your life may not always be fun. Who wants to take out the garbage, anyway, when "forgetting" results in someone else doing the nasty chore? You're trading in a moment of laziness (physical and emotional), then scrambling to make up for it, after the fact—wasting time and precious mental resources. You're also acting out in a passive-aggressive way to your partner, colleague, or friend. By "forgetting" your anniversary, are you really saying that the event (or your marriage) really doesn't matter to you? Is "forgetting" to attend an important meeting a way of telling your boss you're dissatisfied with your job?

Taking the reins by making a conscious effort to remember things, on the other hand, means being honest with your true self and with the people around you. Almost everyone has the ability to be organized and keep things under control. It's just that you—along with thousands of others—often choose to take the "easy" (Read: *lazy*) way out.

But if staying on top of appointments and responsibilities truly eludes you, here are a few tips to get you started:

➤ Keep a day planner, and live with it. Keep it under your pillow if you have to. Write down every appointment you schedule, every idea you have, and every item you want to purchase. Document absolutely everything you may need to remember later.

➤ Become a list-maker. Lists, lists, and more lists. Shopping lists, lists of expenses, to-do lists, chore lists, lists of birthdays you need to remember, lists of special events. Post them on bulletin boards, refrigerators, front doors, car mirrors. And always have something to write on and something to write with wherever you go.

➤ Buy a case of Post-It notes. Use them. Many a computer screen, calendar, car dashboard, and bulletin board are gaily bedecked with these multicolored slips of paper, each bearing a crucial tidbit of must-remember information.

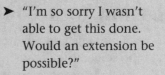

One Day at a Time
Consider these alternatives to everyday "white lies." They're called "the truth!"

➤ "I'm so sorry I wasn't able to get this done. Would an extension be possible?"

➤ "I hate to admit this, but I did forget. How can I make it up to you?"

➤ "That's an interesting look for you. I wouldn't have thought of it."

➤ "I've planned my time badly. Could we possibly postpone? I promise to make it next time!" (But that means you really *do* have to make it next time.)

➤ At the beginning of each day, before you head off to your busy life, stop, sit, breathe, and take a moment to relax. Then slowly go over your day in your mind—using, of course, your appointment book for reference. What's happening today? What do you need to do? Whom do you need to see or call? What's crucial and what could you leave for another day? At the end of the day, just before bed, review your list. Did you accomplish everything? Briefly consider what you need to do tomorrow. Relax some more. Breathe. Now get a good night's sleep!

➤ Yoga, meditation, deep breathing, and other types of relaxation techniques can actually help to clear your mind and focus your thoughts more effectively. Try it.

A New Angle

If you're one of the many people who thinks memory gets worse as you get older, think again. Memory disintegrates out of disuse, not (in most cases) due to age. "Use it or lose it" couldn't be truer when it comes to your memory.

Losing Your Cool

"I don't lie and I don't forget things!" you may be growling, impatiently. "Can we get on to something useful?" Ah, we see now who you are. You're the one with the temper. Yes, anger is as dangerous a form of miscommunication as lying, and you may often lie (by saying things you don't really mean) mostly when you're angry.

Anger erodes self-esteem and destroys trust. Like lying and forgetting, anger results in a failure to communicate and can damage a relationship. When you're angry, or even irritated, you aren't thinking clearly or rationally. Things seem darker, less reasonable, and less tolerable to the angry person than they do to the same person in good-mood mode. Anger also allows you to avoid discussing what's really bothering you in a sane, measured, and constructive way.

Are you an angry person by nature? Do you use anger to avoid stress or other emotions that make you feel uncomfortable? Are you too angry for your own good? To help you get a handle on your anger habits, take the following quiz:

Cold Turkey

In some cases, frequent anger and/or irritation can be a sign of depression. If you can't seem to control your anger no matter how hard you try, and if you often feel despairing or that life is meaningless, consider seeing your doctor. Depression is highly treatable.

1. Do you often get angry enough to slam doors or throw things?   *Yes*____   *No*____

2. Are you unable to let go of an aggravating incident and continue to get angry whenever you think about it?   *Yes*____   *No*____

3. If someone has more than ten items in an eight or under checkout line, does the thought of violence occur to you?   *Yes*____   *No*____

4. Do you flash your lights, honk your horn, or perform some ritualistic gesture when someone cuts you off in traffic?   *Yes*___   *No*____

170

5. Does your pulse climb whenever you're challenged in an argument?
   *Yes*____ *No*____

6. If a friend is late for an event, do you plan the angry words you're going to spew while you wait? *Yes*____ *No*____

If you can answer "yes" to more than one or two of these questions, it's time to get a handle on your anger. Clearly, keeping a positive attitude is important for achieving your goals and maintaining successful relationships. So how can you stop from getting so gosh-darned irritated all the time? Your first step is to admit your feelings, and then try to explore what's behind them. You may be surprised to discover that the object of your rage is not always the underlying problem. Here are a few tips to help you begin to manage your anger:

➤ If something someone does makes you angry on a regular basis, talk to the source of your anger when you aren't feeling angry. Ask how you can fix the situation so you won't fly off the handle and say something you don't mean.

➤ Imagine yourself in the other's person's shoes. How might they be feeling? Looking at the situation from another point of view can help you see it more objectively (and more empathetically, too!).

➤ Leave the situation for awhile until you cool off.

➤ When possible, avoid people and situations that irritate you. Don't go to that particular party or restaurant if you dislike the people or the service. Take an alternate route to work if traffic is bumper-to-bumper. Ask if you can move to a different cubicle in the office if a coworker drives you crazy.

➤ Before you utter one single word, even as you feel the gall just beginning to rise, take a minute to breathe deeply, relax, and think about the best way to handle the situation. Sometimes a slight pause is all it takes to avert an explosion.

Another tip is, of course, to keep a Daily Anger Management Log (set up just like your Truth Log or Daily Habit Log) so you gain a better understanding of what triggers your temper flare-ups and the solutions that help you better manage your emotions. Remember, you may well find that you're taking out your anger on the people you love the most, and failing to directly address the source of your frustration.

What We Have Here Is a Failure to Communicate

Many negative behavioral habits can be reduced to one problem: A failure to communicate effectively and honestly. We've given you some tips for overcoming some specific bad habits involving a lack of communication. Let's look at the major sources of failures to communicate.

Overcoming Stress

Many people in their 40s and 50s complain of increased forgetfulness, and fear they're exhibiting the first symptoms of Alzheimer's disease. Most of the time, however, the source of sudden forgetfulness can be directly traced to stress. Think about it. When you have too much going on at once, do you start to scramble your words, spell things incorrectly, miss appointments, or forget to pick up the kids? Being under stress is like driving a car with an oil leak or a bad carburetor. You aren't running efficiently, and your brain isn't operating at its full potential.

A New Angle

Alzheimer's disease is not a normal part of aging. It affects a small but significant percentage of older Americans, and only a handful of them are under 50 years of age. Most are over 65. Only 5 to 6 percent of older people suffer from Alzheimer's disease or some other related dementia, but that translates to three to four million Americans.

Even if you are approaching or withdrawing from your 40s and 50s, stress can still cause you to forget, as well as to lose your temper. When you're under stress, everything seems more difficult, even insurmountable.

So how do you practice sound stress management?

➤ Exercise regularly. Amazingly, when you make time for exercise, you'll feel like extra time has been added to your day, not taken away.

➤ Cut down on caffeine and sugar. (See Part 3, "Resist Those Cravings.")

➤ Try yoga, meditation, or deep breathing, even if for only a few minutes a day. (Try *The Complete Idiot's Guide to Yoga* to help get you started.)

➤ Don't overplan. Learn to say "no" when your calendar is getting too full. You have the right to keep some of your time for yourself.

➤ Get enough sleep. Easier said than done? Don't nap during the day, don't consume any caffeine after noon, and schedule your day so it actually comes to an end at some point—preferably before midnight!

Your Itchy Trigger Finger

Sometimes, despite your best intentions, things happen to spark your habits back into action. Knowing what triggers your habits will help you to avoid those triggers, which is a lot easier than stopping the behavior once it's started again. Keeping a journal every day to analyze what you're doing before you become angry, start to procrastinate big-time, or slip into your next fib will help you to identify your triggers. Structure your journal something like the following.

MONDAY	What I Did	HABIT ALERT!	How I Felt Afterwards	I COULD have...
Morning	Got the mail—seven bills!	Screamed at the dog	Really guilty—poor Fido didn't wrack up my debts!	Immediately balanced my checkbook and paid what bills I could so they wouldn't be sitting around.
Afternoon	Was feeling overwhelmed about those bills.	Forgot to meet Mom for lunch; when she called, I said I was getting the flu.	Bad about lying, and sad that I missed a free lunch!	Been organized enough to write the lunch date on a calendar that I check at the beginning of each day.
Evening	Ate too much for dinner; felt like I had the stomach flu after all!	Put off exercising again because I felt too full and fat.	Too full and fat.	Forgone a second helping of spaghetti, skipped the cheesecake, then taken a nice evening walk with the dog.
How'd I Do Today?	Not too well. I pretty much indulged all my bad habits. Now I see what I could have done though. I'm committed to try harder tomorrow. I'm worth it! (I'm feeling better already!)			

Talking About It

The very best outlet you have is the one you've used only to your disadvantage so far: Your own mouth. Talking with family, friends, even a therapist, openly and honestly, about the challenges you face is the best way to gain control over your communication problems. Just getting your feelings off your chest and receiving a little moral support is great for your resolve. No one is an island, after all! Let your loved ones lend you a hand, and then you'll know how to do the same for them someday—with honesty and love. (Talk about a great way to subvert miscommunication!)

The Least You Need to Know

➤ Depending on lying, forgetting, or expressions of anger to avoid stress is a very bad habit.

➤ There are few instances when lying doesn't undermine relationships or your own sense of integrity.

➤ Communication bad habits help hide your true feelings.

➤ Managing stress and understanding your triggers will help you win the battle against your bad habit.

➤ The truth will set you free!

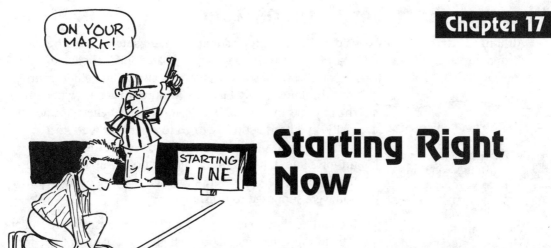

Chapter 17

Starting Right Now

In This Chapter

➤ Identifying your procrastination habits

➤ The motivations behind procrastination

➤ Being on time and in control

How long did you put off reading this chapter? You've known it was here since you read the Table of Contents, and we even alerted you to its presence chapters ago. Did you take the proverbial bull by the horns and plunge right in, or did you meander through information about bad habits you *don't* have just to avoid this moment for as long as possible?

Don't worry. We understand. Procrastination is a common, but tough, nut to crack. No doubt, though, it affects some parts of your life more than others: Are you great at keeping the carpet vacuumed but lousy at working on your doctoral dissertation? Can you write a short story at the drop of a hat, but when it comes to buying gifts, you spend every Christmas Eve at the mall just as it's closing, banging on the doors and begging security guards to let you come in? Maybe you never put off anything that can be done at work, but when you have to take work home with you, the television becomes a far more compelling focus for your attention. Or maybe, no matter how hard you try, you just can't get anywhere on time.

When You Can't Get There on Time

Although it isn't normally considered classic procrastination, being late is, nonetheless, a form of procrastination, and a particularly annoying form at that. Some people are chronically late. You know who you are! (And so does everyone else.) You delude yourself into thinking it only takes six minutes to get anywhere in the city, at any time of day. You sincerely believe (or do you really?) you can get ready to go to a party or work in 10 minutes. And you always forget until you're already 30 minutes late that you need at least another 30 minutes to finish the dessert you were supposed to bring or the report you were supposed to finish.

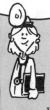

Strictly Speaking

To be **passive-aggressive** is to try to get things you want or control people without actively doing so. When you were a teen-ager, did your mother ever say, "Oh, these groceries are so heavy and I'm so tired! If only someone would help me!" instead of asking you straight out to pitch in and help? Whether it worked or not, your mother performed a classic passive-aggressive move!

It could be that you're chronically late because you're bad at scheduling your time—and we'll give you plenty of tips for better organizing that part of your life. But being late often stems from other motivations: You may also be expressing *passive-aggressive* and controlling behavior. Face it: When you're late, other people suffer. They wait for you, or if they're unlucky enough to be going along with you, they end up late too, even though they were ready to go on time.

Are you chronically late because you're simply disorganized, or are your delays more like power plays? Check all the following that apply:

❏ I'm only late for things I don't really want to do.

❏ People often get irritated at me for being late, but that's their problem—they're just being perfectionists.

❏ I don't mind all that much being late all the time. It's just the way I am.

❏ If I had more control over my life, I wouldn't be late so often.

❏ I feel really guilty when I'm late.

❏ I'm consistently late for just about everything. People know it and expect it. Why change?

❏ If I was more organized, I wouldn't be late so often.

❏ I absolutely hate being late. Late people are so irresponsible—but I just can't seem to get there on time!

If you checked more than two of the first four statements, you may be using your tardiness to control others and to exert power. If you checked more than two of the second four boxes, you're probably merely disorganized and unmotivated. If you checked more than two in both halves of the list, your tardiness is probably due to both controlling behavior and disorganization.

Yes, You! A Procrastination Self-Test

Before we go any further, let's figure out whether you really have a procrastination problem or not. If you don't, you can skip the rest of this chapter! But if you do (and we're guessing you do because most of us do), you'll be able to proceed with a personal procrastination profile in mind. Pick the one best answer to each of the following questions:

1. You're late for work:

    (a) Never.

    (b) About once a week.

    (c) Every day.

2. Organized people:

    (a) Must be a little obsessive.

    (b) Are to be admired and revered.

    (c) Are just like you—you're one of them!

3. Cleaning your home is:

    (a) A task you adore because it allows you to organize, organize, organize.

    (b) A task you merely endure, but perform on a fairly regular basis.

    (c) A task you avoid like the plague.

4. You would most like to spend your day off:

    (a) Organizing photographs into dated and alphabetized archives.

    (b) Catching up on your soaps and ordering Chinese food.

    (c) Relaxing a little, then performing some house-cleaning tasks and getting caught up on some work for the office.

5. When faced with a difficult assignment your boss insists you finish over the weekend, you tend to:

    (a) Color coordinate the file folders, spell check the instructions, then work all night so you can fax it to your boss on Sunday.

    (b) Hide the folders under a pile of laundry.

    (c) Break down the task into manageable segments, play with your kids for an hour, then knuckle down and get started.

6. When it comes time to renew your driver's license, you:

    (a) Plan a vacation.

    (b) Organize your next day off so you'll be able to get your car serviced at a nearby station while you're at the DMV, and then on the way home, be able to pick up the dry-cleaning. And all three weeks before your license expires.

    (c) Grit your teeth and get to the DMV on your next day off.

7. You're supposed to call your mother-in-law to discuss holiday plans. Instead you:

    (a) Clean the cat box, wash the windows, clip your toenails—anything but pick up that phone.

    (b) Make your spouse call her, but with a prepared list of topics to be settled.

    (c) First go through your Martha Stewart holiday planner, make out a complete guest list, prepare the entire menu, then call her exactly at the time you prearranged.

8. Your home office is:

    (a) Neat, organized, and efficient. You've constructed cubbyholes and stacked trays for all possible categories of documents you might encounter.

    (b) Somewhere under an avalanche of paper.

    (c) Mostly functional, though papers do get out of hand sometimes, and you have to devote some serious time to organizing every couple of weeks.

9. Television is:

    (a) A nice distraction while you do an unpleasant task like folding the laundry.

    (b) Your primary avoidance tool, sucking up your energy and time.

    (c) What's a television?

10. Your personal motto is:

    (a) Whenever. Maybe.

    (b) Don't put off until tomorrow what you can *reasonably and sanely* do today.

    (c) There's a time for every purpose under heaven, and that time is NOW.

Score your test as follows:

1. A-1, B-2, C-3	**6.** A-3, B-1, C-2
2. A-3, B-2, C-1	**7.** A-3, B-2, C-1
3. A-1, B-2, C-3	**8.** A-1, B-3, C-2
4. A-1, B-3, C-2	**9.** A-2, B-3, C-1
5. A-3, B-1, C-2	**10.** A-3, B-1, C-2

If you scored between 10–15, you certainly don't have a problem procrastinating, but you may have a problem obsessing. You're so neat, organized, and efficient that it sometimes rules your life. Your habits are more in line with those we discuss in Chapter 20, "Your Very Personal, Personal Space."

If you scored between 16–24, you procrastinate like most of us: some of the time. Procrastination is often a problem for you, though not in every area of your life. The trick is to find where you procrastinate and tackle that particular area. For example, you may never turn in an assignment late or miss an appointment, but you really have trouble getting motivated to wash those dishes!

If you scored between 25–30, you're a procrastinator extraordinaire. This chapter is written with you in mind. You may use your nature as an excuse, thinking you're simply easygoing and can't stand the tedium of mindless chores or irrelevant busywork, but you've got to realize these too are a part of life for everyone. No one likes scrubbing baked-on lasagna from a pan or balancing the checkbook, but these chores come with being a responsible human. Later, we provide you with valuable tips on how to cut down on your tendency to procrastinate. In the meantime, it's time to explore some of the reasons getting started might be tough for you.

What's Stopping You

Why on earth *procrastinate*? Why not just get the job done, get there on time, and move on with your life? Isn't being passive-aggressive a pretty round-about way to accomplish things, and wouldn't life be simpler and more efficient without procrastination? Certainly. But our minds are sometimes too complex for our own good, and lots of things can get in the way of behavior that's sensible.

179

A New Angle

The word "procrastination" comes from the Latin verb *procrastinare*, which combines "pro," meaning "forward motion," with *crastinus*, meaning "belonging to tomorrow."

Remember Phoebe, the procrastinating graphic designer you met in Chapter 6, "Step 2: Evaluate Risks and Benefits"? When she examined her reasons for procrastinating, she discovered they weren't worth the results.

According to the book *Procrastination and Task Avoidance* by J. R. Ferrari and J. L. Johnson, people procrastinate because of one or more of the following mistaken beliefs:

➤ They overestimate how much time they have left to finish a task.

➤ They underestimate how long it will take to complete a task.

➤ They overestimate how motivated they'll be "tomorrow" or at some other time in the future.

➤ They mistakenly believe they must "feel like" doing something to succeed at it.

Do any of these motivations ring true for you? Does Friday seem an awfully long time away when you're given an assignment on Monday? Think again. Do you think you'll be able to zip through a complex task (even though it took you three days of hard work to complete a similar task the last time)? And the "I'll be SO much more efficient and creative TOMORROW" is a remarkably undermining procrastination trap. (Remember Scarlett, the "I'll think about it tomorrow" queen?!) Once again, we're going to ask you to keep your Daily Habit Log (with some dedication this time—don't put it off!). Track the way you cope, or fail to cope, with your daily responsibilities. See what motivates your procrastination, and weigh the results of your actions against the potential benefits of starting and finishing a task on time. You may find your procrastinating nature has something to do with our old friend Fear.

Fear of Failure

It makes sense to fear failure. Nobody wants to fail, but sometimes this fear can keep us from trying something in the first place. Why start that project your boss assigned you if you know, deep down, that it's just a little over your head? Why not wait until tomorrow to confront your teenager's bad behavior, since you know an unpleasant argument is likely to ensue? If you can't convince yourself you're good enough or motivated enough to handle something, it seems futile even to start.

On the other hand, being afraid to fail doesn't make sense; if your fear holds you back from even attempting a task, failure is inevitable. Teams that don't show up for a game have to forfeit, and to forfeit is still to lose.

And woe to you perfectionists out there! Those of you saddled with a perfectionist nature fear failure more than anyone, and you may be the worst procrastinators of all.

If you're such a perfectionist that you aren't even sure what's realistic, ask a few close friends to help you develop some goals. (Pick your non-perfectionist friends, please, or it will be the blind leading the blind!)

> **Strictly Speaking**
> **Perfectionism** is a self-defeating behavior that involves having excessively high, unrealistic standards for yourself (and maybe others). In effect, perfectionism discourages you from pursuing a task because the realistic part of you knows you won't be able to meet your own standards.

Are you a perfectionist? Answer these questions to find out.

➤ Are you always dissatisfied after completing a task because you think you didn't do a good enough job?

➤ Are you often late at completing projects even though you start them on time because you keep trying to redo them until they're perfect?

➤ Do you feel that anything less than a perfect grade or evaluation means you're a failure?

If you answered "yes" to any of the above, you suffer from perfectionism. Mild cases can push you to higher performance levels, but consider severe cases akin to a chronic disease. Let this book be the first step in your treatment plan! Then try the following anti-perfectionist tips:

➤ Set realistic goals based on what you've accomplished in the past, not on what you think you should be able to accomplish or what someone else has accomplished.

➤ Practice doing something in an acceptable—but not perfect—manner, just to save time. Did the world end? Nope! Sometimes, less than 100 percent effort on less important projects is necessary to get everything done.

➤ Focus on performing the task, not only on the end result. Remember to take joy in the process, while considering the goal as necessary but secondary.

➤ Whenever you start to feel stressed, take it as a warning that you're probably expecting too much of yourself. Reevaluate your goals.

➤ Force yourself to make mistakes once in awhile. Did the world end? Nope! Instead of berating yourself, think about what you learned from the mistake.

➤ Remember that there's no such thing as "all or nothing." "Some" is a perfectly acceptable word in the English language, and so is the phrase, "good enough."

A New Angle

According to a 1997 study, up to 70 percent of college students admit they procrastinate regularly.

Fear of Success

Fear of success? Who would be afraid of success? It's what we all want, isn't it? Well, not necessarily. Most of us think we want to be successful, but if success gets too close, some of us run the other way. Why? On her popular talk show, Rosie O'Donnell once said that when she was at her lowest weight, she found herself talking to a man and realized he was flirting with her. Her next stop? The local ice cream shop to alleviate the anxiety the situation provoked in her. Sometimes being overweight or stuck in middle management or "working on a novel" is a lot more comforting and a lot less stressful than having a beautiful body, running the company, or being, say, Stephen King. We'd like to think we'd like the rewards of success (imagine Stephen King's bank account), but what about the changes (good and bad) that come with it?

Fear of success is probably more common than most people realize. Consider the following questions to determine if you might be afraid to succeed:

➤ Are you afraid that making lots of money means you're an adult, with adult responsibilities?

➤ Do you think if you're successful, people will be more likely to take advantage of you?

➤ Do you long to be at a healthier weight or in better shape, but resist all efforts to actually get there?

➤ Do you sometimes feel like you're an impostor—as if you've fooled everyone around you into believing you can be an adult and do the job you do?

Success, especially when it's sudden, will certainly change your life, and people tend to resist change. But if you never take any risks or strive to be better, you may come to the end of your life regretting that you never finished that novel or ran that marathon or started your own business. What's the worst that could happen if you succeed? If you lose friends, they weren't good friends to begin with. If you strike it rich, you can use your money for good. If you look and feel great, you'll probably live a lot longer, not only because you are healthy but because you have a good self-image and lots of confidence. But if you fail to put effort into losing weight you'll never get there. Success is great! So stop procrastinating and start reaching for that brass ring.

Feeling Overwhelmed

Stress. It's always just around the corner, ready to rear its ugly head, isn't it? Stress is certainly a major cause of procrastination for many, from working parents to single executives, even to college students. When you've got a full class load and seven tests on Monday, you may very well end up at the ice cream parlor with Rosie.

When you're under a great deal of stress, the first thing to do—before you even start to get to work—is to tackle the stress. Take a long, hot bath. Do some yoga. Listen to relaxing music. Get a massage. Take a nap (a short one—don't sleep the day away in despair!). Then, when you're feeling more calm, make a list, prioritize your work, and start with the most crucial task. Stay calm, and don't try to work when your head is about to explode. You don't need a mess like that to clean up!

One Day at a Time
If you're having trouble starting an unpleasant chore, play a game with yourself. Pretend you're competing with a cleaning service to see who can clean a living room faster. Imagine that you're being chased by a mob of adoring fans who want your autograph instead of merely jogging. Can you think of 10 ideas for that presentation before your competition does?

Time Management Missteps

No secret agendas, no hidden feelings of resentment or anger, no fear of failure. Some people procrastinate simply because they don't know how to manage their time effectively. Here's a study guide we call "The Ten Commandments of Time Management." Memorize it. Live it.

The Ten Commandments of Time Management

I. **Thou Shalt Not Depend on External Influences to Accomplish Tasks.** Don't think that work will miraculously get done in two weeks simply because you've got a two-week deadline. The work has to come from you.

II. **Thou Shalt Not Believe Thou Must Do It All.** You can't do everything, even if people expect it. Only your own expectations matter, so set reasonable goals. (See Chapter 8 for more information on goal-setting.)

III. **Thou Shalt Learn How to Say No.** Don't want to serve on that committee? Don't want to contribute cookies to that bake sale for the fifth time this month? Don't want to watch your neighbor's six kids for the weekend? Just say no, and watch how your to-do list shrinks.

IV. **Thou Shalt Abandon Certain Tasks for the Sake of Thy Sanity.** You know those items that have been on your to-do list for months, that you really should do but they aren't urgent enough to warrant action? Cross them off. Really. Maybe another time, when you aren't so overextended, you can add them back. Maybe.

V. **Thou Shalt Master the Art of the List.** Lists save the day.

VI. **Thou Shalt Learn to Delegate.** What're kids for if not to help out around the house? Okay, so that wasn't the main reason you had the cute little duffers, but as long as they're part of the household.... And what're roommates for if not to help you study (as long as you return the favor)? And significant others, well, they're significant because they're partners in life, in work, and in getting stuff done, right? And really, what're cleaning services for if not to hire?

VII. **Thou Shalt Practice Stress Management.** The most comprehensive and well-thought-out list in the world won't do you any good if you clutch it in a trembling hand while crouching in a corner, drooling. If the stress in your life is too much, deal with it. Then tackle the list.

VIII. **Thou Shalt Take Care of Thyself.** Eat right. Get enough sleep. You'll make much better use of the time you have if you're physically at your best. Your brain will work better, too.

IX. **Thou Shalt Not Be Too Rigid.** If you concoct an elaborate schedule that begins something like: 6:00 p.m., arrive home from work. 6:15 p.m., start dinner. 6:30 p.m., go through mail. 6:45 p.m., put in a load of laundry. 7:00 p.m., eat your salad. 7:10 p.m., move on to the main course, etc., you're being too rigid. You'll never be able to stick to the exact schedule every single day, and once you break it, you may just give up.

X. **Thou Shalt Prioritize.** Know what has to be done, what should be done, and what you'd like to get done. If you get through the day getting done what has to be done, consider yourself a success. Remember when you didn't even get that far? What a master of time management you have become!

Plain Old Laziness

Don't get us wrong. A certain amount of laziness, at certain times in our lives, is perfectly natural, and actually helpful in relieving stress. But if you're chronically lazy, you're holding yourself back, living only in the moment. When you're in your 60s—and that's something you *won't* be able to put off!—do you want to look back on a long life full of television and two-for-one margaritas? Maybe that doesn't sound so bad right now, but let's just say you only get one life. Suddenly, boom, it's over. What did you do with it? Did you make the most of it? Did you live, or did you just sort of hang out?

Laziness is a hard habit to kick, and procrastination's best friend. Try these tips to kick the habit:

➤ **Get more exercise.** You'll probably have so much energy the very thought of sitting all night in front of sitcoms with a big plate of super nachos will sound tedious and fairly unpleasant. And remember, exercise doesn't have to mean the gym or a marathon: Take a walk around the block after dinner, take the stairs instead of the elevator, turn on some music while you clean and really boogy down!

➤ **Get a buddy.** Enlist an energy-boosting friend to help motivate you. Sure, he or she will watch a couple of videos you'll both enjoy, but may also encourage a walk or quick game of one-on-one during intermission!

➤ **Cut down on sugar and fat.** Stick to energy-boosting low-fat protein and complex carbohydrates as much as possible.

➤ **Establish clear and reasonable goals.** If you keep your goals clearly in mind, and keep reminding yourself why you want to achieve them, you may be able to motivate yourself.

Stop Procrastinating!

All right, time to get down to basics by reviewing and summarizing the very best ways to avoid procrastination, no matter what its cause. Not every trick will work for you, so feel free to try a few on for size. Soon enough, you'll find the best combination for your particular procrastination profile.

Breaking Big Tasks into Little Ones

This old stand-by works great when a task seems too daunting to tackle. If you've got to research a complex subject, break it down into smaller ideas first, then work on one at a time. If your bedroom closet is hiding colonies of raccoons or still contains remnants from your 1970s wardrobe, spend 30 minutes a day sorting through it—tossing out anything you haven't worn in two years—until it's done. And don't waste time getting each step perfect—the point is to keep progressing.

Making Lists

"I get it, I get it!" you're saying by now. "Enough already with the lists!" But lists are the best way—often the *only* way— to remember everything you need to do. They also let you see how much you've accomplished as you cross off each item.

Rewarding Yourself

Life is full of bargains, so why not keep on bargaining with yourself once you've reached adulthood? If you clean the kitchen before you go to sleep, you get to take a 30-minute bubble bath with candles and classical music. If you finish your report tonight, you get to go out for dinner. If you lose that extra 10 pounds, you get to buy a new pair of jeans—in a new size! Whenever an unpleasant task presents itself, before you make one single excuse to put it off, make yourself a deal. You just might be willing to get right to work.

The Motivation Factor

Getting motivated is really tough when all you want to do is roll over and go to sleep or channel surf or eat a quart of Ben & Jerry's. But motivation is the key to procrastination eradication. Clear goals and a sense of who you are and what you can be are perhaps the best motivators of all. And don't forget friends to encourage you, good health to energize you, and confidence to propel you.

Tomorrow Is Another Day

You mean, even after that pep talk, you procrastinated again today? Don't punish yourself or you'll backslide. Chalk it up to experience. Call it the "whoops factor." Then move on. Tomorrow really is another day, and that's not an excuse to procrastinate (again, remember Scarlett?), it's an excuse to start fresh. Even if you made just a little progress today (it only took you 30 minutes instead of all night to get started on scrubbing that mildew ring or making that call to Aunt Helga), that's great. In fact, that's just wonderful!

The Least You Need to Know

➤ Procrastination is not being able to get things done or get somewhere on time.

➤ Fear of failure or success, stress, lack of good time management, and laziness can all contribute to procrastination.

➤ Breaking down big tasks, making lists, and rewarding yourself can all help to waylay procrastination.

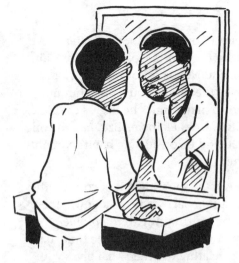

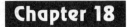

Chapter 18

Establishing Emotional Integrity

In This Chapter

➤ Relationship habits: Out with the bad, in with the good

➤ Overcoming family patterns

➤ How to stop sabotaging love

➤ Getting along with anyone, including yourself!

Humans are social animals. We aren't like spiders, spinning complex webs or constructing elaborate underground burrows without thought or need of another spider dropping by to trade housefly recipes or web-building tips with us. Everything we do exists within a social framework and is done for our own benefit and for the benefit of those around us. Humans thrive on communication, a social network that keeps us engaged with one another. We come to know and identify ourselves through our relationships.

Good relationship habits can only foster productivity, happiness, and good communication. Bad relationship habits—well, have you tuned in to *Melrose Place* lately? Bad relationship habits can wreak havoc. If *your* life's starting to feel as melodramatic as a prime-time soap, it's time to take a break from the action and figure out what's *really* going on.

Did I Do That?

A lot of us do things and don't even realize the impact of our behavior until later—or until someone else points it out to us. Did you ever see the *Seinfeld* episode where Elaine keeps hanging up when she calls her friend, Noreen, and Noreen's boring, chit-chatty significant other answers the phone and won't shut up? Elaine cuts the man off so many times he begins to think Noreen's having an affair. Does Elaine realize *she's* the one who's really got the bad and inconsiderate habit? Not until Jerry points it out to her.

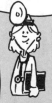

Strictly Speaking
A **mediator** is a person who acts as an intermediary or conciliator between two or more people. There are both legal mediators, who may help two people settle a legal dispute outside the court system, and psychological mediators (counselors or therapists) who help troubled couples and families work out emotional issues.

When a situation seems to be spiraling out of control, the first thing to do is take a step back and consider whether your own actions may be contributing to the problem without your conscious awareness. At the same time, foster a sense of objectivity in relating to others that gives you some room to observe what's happening without being drawn in by the heat of the moment. Use your Daily Habit Log to record your feelings and thoughts when you interact with someone with whom you've got a difficult or challenging relationship. Examine the log to see if consistent triggers, expressions, or outcomes emerge as a pattern in your encounters. What you find may help you take a new, more constructive approach.

Strictly Speaking
Empathy is the ability to look past for a moment what *you're* thinking and feeling, to be able to understand feelings and viewpoints, which may be very different from yours, that are held by someone else.

Mediators use communication techniques to help people become more aware of how their behavior is affecting others, and to reveal relationship sabotage. Say you're involved in a dispute over a repair with your landlord. You've been withholding rent because a leaking roof hasn't been fixed for three months, it's rainy season, and the landlord's nowhere to be found. Your landlord insists you never agreed to the contractor's schedule and that you resent it if anyone tries to come into the house to look around. Who's right?

An effective mediation technique is to have one person tell his or her story without stopping and without interruption, say within a five-minute time limit. Then, the opposing person restates that point of view in different words. Both people get a chance to air their views and have them repeated by the other person; they're forced to "wear each other's shoes" (or, in this example, galoshes!). *Empathy* goes a long way to creating understanding and working toward solutions that acknowledge *both* points of view.

The Top 10 Things You Need from People in Your Life

Admitting that you need other people isn't a sign of weakness. It's simply a fact of life. But for some of us, learning the give-and-take dance of adult relationships is harder than it is for others. Knowing what you need from people and what they'll need from you in return is an important step toward achieving emotional integrity.

1. **Support.** Without encouragement and positive reinforcement, self-doubt and fear can creep in and do their undermining work.

2. **Trust.** Trust allows you to reveal your vulnerable side, your secret hopes and fears. Constructive trust makes us stronger as we help others and receive help from them. But trusting too much, too little, or in the wrong people is a common bad relationship habit.

3. **Touch.** Humans need physical contact with one another, and rear-ending someone's car or exchanging mushy but anonymous e-mail messages don't count on that score. We need to hug, shake hands, pat each other on the back, kiss. It doesn't hurt to brush each other's hair, smooth each other's brows, or exchange foot rubs either. Touch makes us feel valued and alive.

4. **Laughter.** If you can laugh at life's ups and downs, you're on the road to putting almost any situation into a perspective where good solutions can be found.

5. **Intimacy.** Going hand in hand with trust, intimacy allows us to explore who we are and to reach toward the people we love. Without it, our relationships lack a richness that comes with letting ourselves be known.

6. **Communication.** It sounds obvious, but you can't have a relationship with someone if you can't communicate. True communication means being able to say what you mean in a way that allows other people to understand you, and being able to listen to others with an open mind, a loving heart, and your full attention.

7. **Community.** Feeling a sense of responsibility to family, neighborhood, state, and country is too much neglected in today's fast-paced society. Volunteering one night a week can help us remain aware of our connection to a greater community—whether it's helping a son or daughter with homework or visiting elders at a local senior center.

8. **Sharing.** Support groups such as Alcoholics Anonymous and Weight Watchers are so popular because they allow members to share their experiences. The other people participating in the group truly understand what you're going through. Just knowing that others are in the same boat can help give you the courage and the strength to row yourself to shore.

191

9. **Sex.** The urge for sex is as natural as the urges to eat and to sleep. Taking responsibility for your sexuality with maturity and compassion can help you develop healthy sexual relationships based on emotional integrity.

10. **Love.** The need for love may be biological and it may be cultural, but it's inarguably a need. Some of us have love dropped in our laps, while others have to work for it, but it's a goal worth a lifetime of effort. We might even venture to say that love is the whole point of being human.

A New Angle

The third week of every July is World Hug Week (July 13–19 in 1998). World Hug Week was begun to promote unconditional acceptance. Promoters encourage people all over the world to hug at least three people per day during hug week, then ask those three to hug three others. (Please ask permission before hugging anyone who might not respond with warmth!)

The Fine Art of Sharing

Derived from the Latin word *communicare* meaning "to share," communication is the process by which we exchange information, ideas, and feelings. It's the essence of all human interaction and the basis upon which individual relationships are built, business transactions conducted, and societies formed. Regrettably, the kinds of qualities we need to communicate effectively—patience, attention, and empathy—are in pretty short supply these days. But they're just what you need if you're trying to form healthier, more satisfying relationships. We could write a book on developing more effective communication skills, but in the meantime, here are a few tips to get you started:

➤ **Pay attention.** When you're conversing with a friend or family member, reduce distractions. Shut off the television, close the office door, choose a quiet restaurant. Make eye contact and watch your partner's body language to pick up non-verbal cues and messages.

➤ **Stop interrupting and finishing others' thoughts.** This communication bad habit is a sure-fire way to alienate the people in your life. Slow down. Listen. Take a deep breath. Ask the person speaking if she or he is finished before you break in. And don't feel you have to fill every second with conversation.

➤ **Break unhealthy patterns.** Do you often take the role of "victim" in your relationships, assigning blame to others for your problems? If so, make a list of your accomplishments and successes. Every time you start to complain or blame, recount one of your triumphs instead. Or are you a "controller" who needs to manage every aspect of your relationship? If that sounds like you, try relinquishing one chore, activity, or decision every day to a family member, spouse, colleague, or friend.

Developing better communication skills may mend some difficult current relationships, as well as help you establish healthy new ones. Since charity begins at home, let's get started by addressing family ties.

All in the Family

No doubt about it, family relationships represent some of the most complex and potentially irritating associations known to humankind. To some extent, you're stuck with your family. You might not have to see them every day, and you might not even like them very much, but your relationship to your family forms an important cornerstone of your life. Even Archie Bunker would agree with that!

"But They Still Treat Me Like I'm 12!"

"Have you gained weight?" your mother asks every time you see her. Or maybe your dad will never in a million years understand why you shunned law school to become a musician. Maybe your brother still disagrees with everything you say. Maybe your sister tells all your secrets. How can you possibly communicate as equals with these people?

It's not easy, that's for sure. It usually means stepping out of the role you're used to playing and standing firm. Replacing your knee-jerk reactions with a more objective and thoughtful approach can go a long way toward revitalizing good family relationships and avoiding bad-habit family patterns that are stagnant and unproductive.

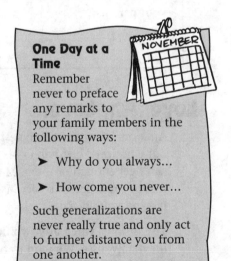

One Day at a Time
Remember never to preface any remarks to your family members in the following ways:

➤ Why do you always...

➤ How come you never...

Such generalizations are never really true and only act to further distance you from one another.

Transforming Family Relationships

We know: It's not your fault. You didn't start it. It's them. But feeling defensive isn't going to get you where you want to go, is it? At least it hasn't so far.

Instead, offer love, respect, and caring wholeheartedly, even if it costs you a little pride and takes a great deal of effort and patience. You'll be amazed at how it will change both the way you feel and, eventually, the way your family treats you.

If you tend to feel frazzled and frustrated after every family visit...	Have a clear goal in mind before you walk in that familiar front door, such as, "Today, I won't criticize anyone" or "Today, I won't take anything personally."
If you tend to flare up in anger whenever anyone provokes you because of all those times in the past...	Decide beforehand to forgive. Forgiveness is the great family healer.
If you tend to criticize and attack certain family members...	Decide not to blame. Blaming is unproductive. If something is bothering you, be straightforward about how you might resolve the problem.
If you feel like an immature teenager or a little kid whenever you are around your parents...	Decide to be a grown-up. Go over your expected behavior beforehand. Think about how you tend to act, then decide what the adult reaction would be. Then do it! (You are a grown-up, after all, remember?)

Love, Ah, Love...

After our families, the biggest relationship challenge—and the one most likely to reveal our emotional bad habits—is our love relationships. Either we can't get rid of someone, or can't get enough of them. Maybe they won't commit, or maybe you push too hard. Or maybe the biggest problem is that, after 10 years of marriage, you no longer share the passion you once did.

The truth is, when any two imperfect people decide to form a relationship, problems will inevitably arise. We tend to tuck our bad habits neatly away when trying to impress someone new, but once your significant other and you become familiar and comfortable, out they spill. Rooting out bad habits before they destroy your relationship is a more productive approach. Read on to find yourself and your negative relationship tendencies.

Inability to Commit

You love her, you think. At least, she loves you, and she sure is a great woman. So why can't you buckle down and commit? Maybe he's everything you always knew you wanted, but now that you've got him, something's missing. Are you a commitment-phobe, or are you simply reacting to a not-quite-right relationship? Answer the following questions to determine your commitment-phobia status.

1. The thought of getting married to your "one and only?!":

   (a) Makes you break out in a cold sweat.

   (b) Seems a natural part of life.

2. You really like the person you just started dating, but you've got a feeling it won't work out because:

   (a) You don't like the way she or he eats cereal in the morning.

   (b) He or she doesn't share your passion for politics/sports/the environment/gourmet cooking/philosophy/jazz, and other things that are really important to you.

3. You've been in a relationship for several years and assume marriage should probably be the next step, but you can't get yourself to mention it because:

   (a) You think if you say the "M" word, the whole wonderful relationship experience will blow up in your face.

   (b) You've felt from the very start that this person didn't really do it for you, even though you're the greatest of friends. You just aren't sure you should end it either, though.

4. You've been hurt before. Your strategy now is:

   (a) To do the hurting first next time.

   (b) To try, try again.

So, where do you fit in? The inability to commit to someone else in a romantic relationship (or in a friendship or professional partnerships) can be caused by a lot of things: a drive for perfectionism, feelings of unworthiness, the need to be free, or fears of being abandoned or becoming too vulnerable to another person. You may also be carrying some baggage left over from childhood: The way your parents related, or failed to relate, could definitely affect your ability and desire to form close ties.

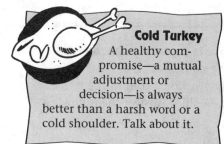

Cold Turkey
A healthy compromise—a mutual adjustment or decision—is always better than a harsh word or a cold shoulder. Talk about it.

There's no easy solution to such entrenched fears and insecurities. But the first step is to simply give it another try! You know that word Captain Picard uses on *Star Trek: The Next Generation* when the crew's about to go off toward a new set of adventures in an unknown and unknowable universe? Engage. Reach out and touch someone, and let him or her touch you back. Whether it's a romance, a friendship, or a business association, you've got to give of yourself—your honesty, your empathy, your humor—in order for the relationship to move forward. If your bad relationship habits are keeping you from engaging the people in your life, you've got some work to do because remaining at an emotional—if not physical—distance will get you nowhere!

Pushing It

Then there are the types who are so desperate for a commitment they push and push long before a relationship is ready. Do you tend to push too hard, too soon? Answer the following questions as openly and honestly as you can:

➤ Do you constantly dwell on the future of your relationship instead of the present?

➤ Do you long for (and often ask for) some symbol or proof of your relationship, such as a ring, a daily declaration of undying love, or (heaven forbid!) a baby?

➤ Do you make assumptions about the future before you've discussed it with your partner, such as, "Oh, we'll be married by this time next year," or "We'll move in together soon"?

➤ Do you feel compelled to give your partner an ultimatum regarding commitment, even though you haven't been together very long?

If you answered "yes" to any of the above, you could be making your potential partner very uncomfortable.

Rather than focusing on what you want (or think you want), try to tune in to what you partner is feeling. You may experience a revelation, and realize he or she isn't the person you thought, and certainly not the one to whom you want to make a serious commitment. Or you may discover that a less aggressive approach may very well get the two of you together quicker than you ever imagined.

Sex: Feast or Famine?

And then there's sex. You want it, you need it, you gotta have it. Or, you used to want it, and it's still nice on occasion, but frankly, you've got better things to do with your time.

Or, you loathe the very thought and honestly wouldn't care if you never had sex again. Or you want it, and just can't get it, because you want it for all the *right* reasons and there isn't an appropriate guy or gal in sight.

Even if you're part of a loving couple, sex can be a problem. You might start out having drastically different sex drives, which only shows how adaptable humans can be when true love is there for support. But in most cases, a once mutually satisfying sexual relationship begins to erode due to very bad communication habits.

If you and your partner have lost interest in sex, try to figure out why. Make a romantic date—complete with candlelight, roses, and—most important—freedom from the kids and other distractions for a few hours. Listen to what your partner has to say, and share your own feelings with honesty. If you can't break down the barriers together, don't give up. Seek the advice and counsel of a qualified therapist. Unfortunately, sex is a subject that too often goes undiscussed out of fear or embarrassment.

People in General

Maybe your problem isn't limited to your family or your love relationships. Maybe it involves other, more peripheral people in your life. Dealing with others is one of the most difficult and most necessary tasks we humans have before us. But some of us tend to deal with most people in certain predetermined, bad habit ways. We're passive-aggressive, we obsess, we idolize, or we assume the worst.

Stalkers Anonymous

Do you allow yourself to be completely consumed by a relationship? Do you obsess about your partner, even to the point of doing things you wouldn't want to admit, such as spying, reading your partner's mail, or even secretly following him or her? Do you call constantly to make sure your partner is where he or she claims? Do you smother your partner with gifts and affection to secure love? After a few weeks or months, do your relationships gradually disintegrate as your partner tries to escape your obsessiveness, and when you sense this, do you step up your efforts even more?

If you sense you might be obsessive about a relationship in your life, try putting everything on hold for a bit—your emotions, your contact with the person, even your hopes and dreams for the relationship. Putting a little time and distance between you and the relationship might help you understand why you feel you need this person so much and what it is you're hoping he or she can offer you. Try to imagine how the person you care about must be feeling about all this obsessive behavior: He or she may be more frightened or annoyed than intrigued or flattered. If you find that you simply cannot control your behavior, consider talking to a therapist who can help you deal constructively with the situation before it really gets out of hand.

The Guru Syndrome

Technically, a guru is a positive force, a sort of spiritual guide who helps you on your quest to "find yourself" or become more spiritually aware. Unfortunately, however, the practice doesn't always match this high ideal. When people find someone they respect or desire to emulate, they may give themselves over completely, relinquishing all sense of self. A true guru can be trusted to guide his or her devotees along a safe and productive path, but too many charismatic people out there are more than happy to take advantage.

Another way to look at this syndrome is in terms of mentorship. A mentor, like a guru, is a wise and trusted teacher. Sure, there are some great mentors ready to help you grow and who want you to succeed. But you have to be a little careful. If someone wants you to invest your money, takes credit for that great budget forecast you formulated for your department at work, or asks you to do anything you feel uncomfortable about or that compromises beliefs that are important to you, be suspicious. (If someone claims to have supernatural powers, this should raise a red flag for sure!)

Remember, no one person can make life "all right" for another person. We all bear the individual responsibility—and positive challenge—for our own well-being and happiness. A true mentor-teacher helps you to do this by fostering your growth and emotional integrity, and won't ever ask you to give up control of your life. Quite the opposite, in fact—a good mentor prods you to take the helm and steer yourself into the future you've imagined and planned for.

Knowing Who's Good for You

So, with all those crazy relatives and non-committal partners and high-pressure pushers and potential stalkers and wanna-be cult leaders out there, who the heck are you supposed to have a relationship with? Calm down, and listen to your heart. Really! Humans do retain some shred of intuition, and deep down, if you're *really* paying attention, you'll probably just know when someone is good for you. Does the person make you feel good about yourself? Does the relationship add energy and vitality to your life? If you can answer "yes" to these two questions, the relationship is certainly on the right track.

Then, it's important to look at your goals for the future to see how the relationship adds to your chances of meeting them. If you're dating someone who wants marriage and children pretty quickly, and you know that you're a long way away from making that kind of commitment, that relationship may not be good for either of you. Knowing what you want, and what it takes to get it, will help you choose your relationships with more wisdom.

If you're still hopelessly confused and don't know what you want or how to take control of your relationships—if you're afraid you might make a good new character on *Melrose*

Place—seek out a therapist or counselor and talk about it with someone who can be objective. It might make all the difference in the world and open up your life to a new way of interacting with others that'll make you feel better about yourself and happier in your life.

The Least You Need to Know

➤ People need people—and that means you!

➤ By changing the way you behave and think, you can take the first step in creating good relationships.

➤ Establishing healthy relationships requires developing a healthy sense of self-esteem and a self-knowledge about your goals and aspirations.

➤ If your relationships are out of control, seeking out a therapist who can give objective counsel may be the best relationship decision you make.

Part 5
Calming Those Compulsions

Part 5 covers the things we feel compelled to do—unconsciously, subconsciously, or quite advertently—over and over again, even if the consequences aren't quite what we're intending.

➤ Is a physical tic, like jaw-clenching or knee-jiggling, driving the people around you crazy?

➤ Does a compulsive need for order—or the opposite need for disorder—prevent you from meeting the personal and professional goals you set for yourself?

➤ Is the fine art of money management completely lost on you? Do you overspend, gamble, or plunge into get-rich schemes, while watching your bank account suffer in the process?

➤ Do you compulsively use the electronic media, specifically the television or the computer—to avoid the stresses and challenges in your life?

If so, read on because we've got some nifty tips to help you relieve your compulsions and channel your new-found energy into more positive behaviors.

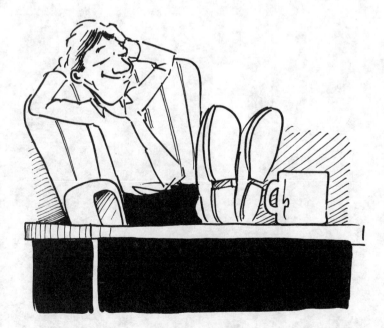

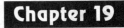

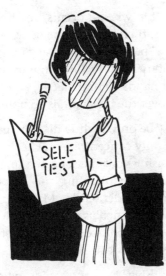

Chapter 19

Identify Your Compulsions

In This Chapter

➤ Understanding your irresistible impulses

➤ Learning tips and techniques to stop compulsive behavior

➤ Putting your energy to better use

Must your desk be in perfect order before you can even begin to work? Or is the reverse true? Like Oscar Madison in *The Odd Couple,* is chaos required to retain mastery over your surroundings?

If you answered yes to either question, your bad habit may fall into the category of a compulsion—a repetitive action you must repeat over and over and over (and over) again. You perform this action (or series of actions) to relieve stress and tension, to control your environment, or to avoid coping with a situation that makes you feel uncomfortable. You are compelled, coerced, irrationally, irresistibly drawn to your bad habit behavior—almost against your own will!

When You Just, Just, Just, Can't Help It

If you're reading this chapter, you probably suspect that your behavior borders on—or spills right over onto—the compulsive. Before you can start to manage your bad habit,

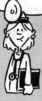

Strictly Speaking
Obsessive-Compulsive Disorder (OCD) involves rigid, ritualistic behavior performed to an extreme degree. People with OCD are in perfectionist pursuit of control—at the expense of openness, flexibility, or efficiency. Preoccupation with rules, lists, and a refusal to delegate are clues to OCD behavior, as are feelings of low self-esteem and powerlessness over the need to perform the rituals.

you need to identify what it is, when it occurs, and how it affects your life. The trick is, there's a fine line between "normal" and "compulsive" behavior. Washing your hands before every meal is a sanitary habit instilled in most of us as children. Washing your hands 30 times a day, and feeling that you have no control over the behavior, is compulsive.

Compulsive behaviors may be only slightly disruptive bad habits, say, when you can only concentrate on checking that spreadsheet if you're using your special green spreadsheet-checking pen, or completely disabling, such as occurs with Obsessive-Compulsive Disorder (OCD). Many extreme obsessive-compulsive behaviors, such as excessive orderliness, are performed by people to reduce stress or forestall or prevent some dreaded event (like death!).

Do you think you're compulsive? Do your friends (who have to wait while you check a dozen times to see if your coffee pot is turned off before you can leave the house) mention the possibility that you have a few bad habits you could lose? Take this self-test and see how compelling your personal compulsions are.

A Compelling Self-Test You Won't Be Able to Resist

For each statement, select the letter that *best* fits you.

1. I twirl my hair:

    (a) Only when I need to create an elegant French braid.

    (b) When I can't think of what else to do with my hands—and I need to do something!

    (c) Occasionally, when I'm under particular stress.

    (d) All the time, so much so that my friends suggest I get a buzz cut.

2. I wash my hands:

    (a) Before every meal or when I touch anything unsanitary.

    (b) When they're really dirty—and not until.

    (c) Before and after every meal, before I leave the house, when I come back home, maybe more often.

    (d) As often as I can—certainly *every* time I touch a doorknob. You can never be clean enough. (Actually, this *is* true for health-care professionals!)

3. I do the dishes:

   (a) After every meal.

   (b) I don't own dishes; I eat out of the can.

   (c) Hardly ever. When I can't find any clean dishes, I scrape off a couple from the dirty stack.

   (d) According to a schedule I keep on a database and update daily.

4. Before I leave the house:

   (a) I double-check that the stove is off.

   (b) I grab my keys and scoot. Sometimes I forget to turn off the stove, but nothing's caught fire yet.

   (c) I'd check the stove if I could find it.

   (d) I check the stove several times, and then call the housekeeper at least twice from the office to double-check.

5. If my boss asks me to stay late:

   (a) I can rearrange my schedule with just two phone calls.

   (b) I can make an excuse in just a few minutes.

   (c) I'll stay, but then my kids will end up having to hitchhike home.

   (d) I'll stay all night and come in early the next morning, for a week if necessary. But first I have to check my home answering machine, 17 times, to make sure I'm not missing anything.

6. I manage my money by paying my bills:

   (a) On time every month.

   (b) Just before I need to use my credit card again.

   (c) Ten minutes before the electricity will be turned off.

   (d) Not often—just ask my credit counselor.

7. My dream of gambling:

   (a) Begins and ends with playing computer Solitaire.

   (b) Involves guessing how much money might be in my checking account at any given moment.

   (c) Is a thrill a minute every Saturday night.

   (d) Has become a nightmare.

8. When I role the dice, it means:

   (a) I'm playing a game of Monopoly with my kids.

   (b) My family better not need me for a few hours because I'll be busy!

   (c) I'll lose more time and money than I can afford, but it feels too good to stop.

   (d) I won't be able to stop until the sun comes up—a week from Thursday.

9. Surfing the Internet is:

   (a) A waste of time—I only look up vital pieces of information on the Web.

   (b) The main reason I don't finish my work on time.

   (c) Taking the place of my relationships with "real" people.

   (d) Sucking the life out of my marriage, and the only thing I look forward to doing all day long.

Scoring: Surprise! No matter what your responses, you're indulging in some type of compulsive—or at least annoying—behavior.

If you answered mostly A's: You're actually a pretty normal, responsible person, someone's who's very organized, orderly, and on an even keel when it comes to relationships. On the other hand, your absolute sanity may be driving your friends and acquaintances right up the wall, especially if you constantly remind them of how well you do everything. Yes, you can usually find what you need, when you need it, but others will wonder just what your organization and efficiency are masking. Have you ever asked yourself that question?

If you answered mostly B's: Your carelessness borders on the compulsive. Although your home life and career may not be seriously affected, your bad habit is probably interfering with your goals and your sense of self-esteem. It may also signal possible codependent behavior: Perhaps you lose things because you know others will help you find them. Or maybe you don't bother to pay your bills on time or clean because you know someone else will do it if you don't. Or perhaps you're compulsive about certain behaviors—like watching television, gambling, or surfing the Internet as a way of avoiding engaging with the people in your life.

If you answered mostly *C's*: You have one or more behaviors that border on the compulsive, and they may well be affecting your ability to function. Read on to find out more about compulsive behaviors and what you can do about them.

If you answered mostly *D's*: Your compulsive need to be in control may be bordering on an obsession. You might want to consider seeing a counselor or therapist who can help you loosen the grip that compulsive behaviors hold on your everyday existence. Read on to find out more about compulsive behaviors and what you can do about them.

One More Time

Now that you've identified the degree of your compulsive behaviors, it's time to start thinking about letting them go. Many perfectly healthy habits stem from the desire to avoid or prevent stressful situations. If you check for your keys before you close your front door, you're avoiding the more unpleasant possibility of locking yourself out. But if you check for your keys *more than once, every time*, your behavior is compulsive. Maybe you don't want to leave home or you may be avoiding issues completely unrelated to the actual behavior.

The key to stopping that "one more time" is to figure out what's triggering it in the first place. It's fine, after all, to make sure the credit card the waitperson returns to you after you pay for a meal is really *yours*—but to check it four times before you leave the restaurant is a little bit more than prudent behavior.

> ### A New Angle
>
> Recent research has suggested that the line between "normal" compulsions and "abnormal" compulsions really is pretty thin. If you always put your pants on right leg, then left leg, you are probably not compulsive. But if you also have to put on your shirt, your sweater, and your coat first right arm, then left arm then you may well have crossed the line.

Your First Time, Redux

Remember when we asked you to remember "your first time" in Chapter 2, "Why You Do the Things You Do"? Think again about the circumstances the first time you performed your compulsive bad habit. What about the first time you updated your databases at 2 p.m.? Maybe as soon as you finished, a caller needed precisely the information you'd just entered. How fortunate you were so efficient—and you swore you'd always be ready no matter what it took. Or perhaps the trigger for your first time was just the opposite: You took the call, but had no idea where the information was. You vowed to never get caught empty-handed again. So now you update your databases three times a day while your in-box piles high with work that requires your more immediate attention.

Triggers for compulsions almost always come from either a *very positive* or a *very negative* experience—and it doesn't have to be your own either. You may have heard a story about someone whose house burned down because he forgot to turn off the iron. Or about someone who got tenure because he could recite thousands upon thousands of lines from the Shakespeare plays.

Whether the trigger is negative or positive, ultimately what compulsions do is allay our fears: our fears of failing, of losing things, of committing to a relationship, of humiliation, or even death. Like any type of bad habit, compulsions have the power to comfort us with their sameness and predictability. But the comfort doesn't alleviate the fear for very long, and so it never fixes the underlying problem.

Once you know what's triggering a compulsion, you can evaluate the risks and benefits associated with it.

A Hard Look at Your Compulsion

Hanna's Risk-Benefit Analysis

My Compulsion: a tidy house

My First Time: when we were selling the house in Virginia

Current Triggers: boredom, stress related to visitors (expected or not)

Risks:
1. Not letting others have their space
2. No time for other activities
3. Feelings of anxiety over normal
4. Use of home by family & friends

Benefits:
1. Always know where things are
2. Enjoyment from cleaning

Look at the "current triggers" in Hannah's risk-benefit analysis. She's trying to be honest, but having a hard time getting to the most destructive trigger: the fear of how others will judge her by the appearance of her house—outside others, not her immediate family, who's actually the ones being harmed by Hannah's compulsive tidiness.

To learn to stop her compulsive behavior, she's going to need to acknowledge that it's the love of those closest to her that matters—not what strangers think. That's where her "first time" comes in: When she was "selling the house in Virginia," it was important to keep the house tidy for strangers. Perhaps it took so long to sell that house, the habit became compulsion. Or perhaps the people who finally bought it complimented her on its tidiness.

But how do you replace a compulsion like this? What are the "rewards" this woman sees that keeps her tidying up her house?

She says she "always knows where things are." Well, there's nothing wrong with that. But what other rewards might she be reaping? *Maybe* she thinks her family perceives her as indispensable because she's the one who always knows where things are.

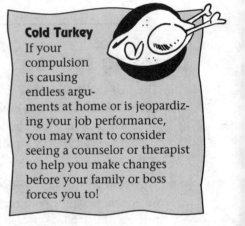

Cold Turkey
If your compulsion is causing endless arguments at home or is jeopardizing your job performance, you may want to consider seeing a counselor or therapist to help you make changes before your family or boss forces you to!

Truth is, her family will perceive her as indispensable whether she tidies the house or not—that's what families are all about, people who are indispensable to each other. Knowing this, maybe she can replace her compulsion with doing other, special, things for her family—like taking them all out for dinner, or tucking little notes into places she knows they'll look. If it's *really* about love, after all, shouldn't the message say so?

A good hard look at *your* compulsions will reveal the same thing—that negative messages can be replaced with positive ones. Fill out your own Risk-Benefit Analysis and begin the soul-searching process that will prepare you for changing your compulsive behavior.

Your Risk-Benefit Analysis

My Compulsion: _____

My First Time: _____

Current Triggers: _____

_____

Risks: _____

_____

Benefits: _____

_____

Learning to Stop

The first step in learning to stop is acknowledging your problem. That's where your risk-benefit chart is going to come in handy. Right there, in black and white, is proof of your behavior, information about what sets it off, and the reasons why you shouldn't indulge. Tape it to your mirror for a few weeks, and see what it tells you about yourself and your bad habit.

The stories about how and why you developed your compulsion aren't always happy ones. You may grit your teeth because you learned early on that your parents wouldn't tolerate "back talk." Or you may not really understand why you chew the end of every pen you lay your hands on, you just know how hard it is to stop today.

The methods for learning to stop are as varied as the compulsive behaviors we acquire. Following, we've provided a list of behaviors and possible methods for modification, but you should think of these as a starting point for your own journey of change, rather than as sure-fire fixes.

Compulsion	Possible Fixes
Cleanliness	Positive Reinforcement
Efficiency	Meditation
Messiness	Positive Reinforcement
Physical Tics	Physical Substitutes; Meditation
Ritual	Positive Reinforcement

Physical Substitutes

Physical substitutes for bad habits usually replace one physical act with another. One interesting, and often successful, substitute for cracking your knuckles, for instance, is snapping a rubber band on your wrist every time you feel the urge to indulge. If you bite your nails, snap your gum, shake your knee, or any of the other "personal" but extremely annoying behaviors, you're manifesting a physical tic that can probably be replaced with a behavior that's less annoying to those around you. Here are some suggestions:

➤ Make an "O" with your thumb and forefinger. (Silent and unobtrusive—especially if you do it in your lap behind a desk.)

➤ Push your tongue against the roof of your mouth. (Ditto.)

➤ Take a deep breath and count to 10. (Yes, it really does work.)

Positive Reinforcement

Positive reinforcement is the catchword in animal training—and for good reason. It's the single most effective method of behavior modification. One of our incorrigibly bad dogs, in fact, learned not to bark at other dogs after just five minutes of positive reinforcement. No dog biscuits. We were impressed. (Actually, we were dumbfounded.)

For a dog, positive reinforcement means saying "Good dog, good dog," every time the dog behaves as you desire. This is coupled with a loud, "No!" when the dog does something less desirable, but you'll soon find there are more "Good dog"s than "No!"s in your home's dog-human communication.

Now, just how would positive reinforcement work for humans? (Could you say "Good dog" and "No!" to yourself? You already know the answer to this.) How do you reward yourself? How do you punish yourself? If the answers involve more bad habits—if you stop cracking your knuckles by overspending or overeating—than you'll end by gaining nothing because bad habits still control you.

One Day at a Time
Positive reinforcement really works—you just have to find the reinforcer that works for you. If you finally decide to work on the troubled relationship you have with your brother, you can set up a system of small rewards—an extra hour at the gym, tickets to a basketball game (maybe even for the two of you)—every time you have a productive conversation. Sooner or later, you'll relate your brother to happier times, which will certainly encourage you to keep the lines of communication open.

Chances are, what makes you happy are the same things that make everybody happy: love, warmth, and respect. The best positive reinforcements, then, are little things you can give yourself (a manicure for a week of no nail-biting, a psychological pat on the back with an internal "good job") or things that others involved in your process of change can offer you (a literal pat on the back, a heart-felt compliment, a bouquet of flowers). Or you can take your successes more public by wearing a special piece of jewelry or a flower in your lapel. If someone asks what the occasion is, you can say, "I'm rewarding myself." You'll probably start a trend.

Meditation

This is not about swamis or gurus or finding your inner child. Meditation is about learning to listen—to yourself.

There are as many meditation methods as there are people who meditate, and only you can decide what method works best for you. Some people find that repeating a mantra, such as "Om," stops the ceaseless audiotape of details our brains play for our continual consideration. Others use deep breathing methods to find their internal rhythm. The key is to relax, clear out the mental clutter, and become mindful of our thoughts and feelings as we experience them, in the moment.

Channeling Your Energy in a New Direction

Just imagine all that energy you put into stacking the canned goods in the kitchen cabinets meticulously by size and contents, arranging those white bathroom towels "just so" so that no one would ever dream of touching (much less using) them, or tapping that toe under the table whenever you take an exam at school. Where else could that energy go? When you let go of your compulsions, you'll find yourself free, flexible, and raring to try new things. Use that energy to join a community action committee (which could use your organizational stamina), volunteer at a local hospital or clinic (which could use your aseptic acumen), or run ten miles (which would make you stronger and more focused). Compulsions, the rituals we perform to gain mastery over our lives, end up doing the opposite; they end up controlling us. One thing in life is certain, everything is uncertain! By embracing the richness of life and all its possibilities, you'll find that the new sense of energy, engagement, and synergy with others that enters your everyday life is far more intriguing and compelling than any compulsion could ever be.

The Least You Need to Know

➤ Compulsions are repetitive actions that help us deal with stress or prevent a dreaded event.

➤ The triggers for compulsive behavior are usually very positive or very negative experiences.

➤ The energy expended on a compulsion can be directed in new and exciting ways that enhance your life instead of limiting it.

➤ Replacement behaviors, such as physical substitution, positive reinforcement, and meditation can help you break compulsive bad habit behaviors.

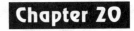

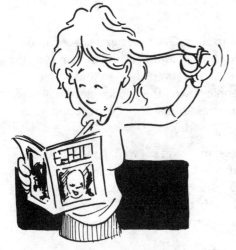

Your Very Personal, Personal Space

What do you do when you're all alone and no eyes of judgment or curiosity are upon you? Do you like to wear the same clothes until they can stand up by themselves? Crack the entire length of your back while you're sitting at the computer? (Feels good, doesn't it? Better than a chiropractor—and cheaper, too!) Play with your chin? Burp? Dare we say it: Pass gas? (Let's be polite.) Do you slurp your cereal and then drink the milk straight from the bowl?

Behind closed doors in the bathroom, do you wash your hands at least 15 times each day; floss *too* much; alternate six types of shampoo and a dozen moisturizers for each body part; or pick your nose?

Well, what you do in your own private sanctuary is one thing. But when those eclectic, quirky, oh-so-you things you do in private start exhibiting themselves—to a not-so-grateful viewing public of family, friends, and possibly even coworkers—your beloved behavior is suddenly revealed to you in all its glorious odiousness as a very ugly and annoying bad habit.

A Close Call

Americans have a lot of personal space, and they like to fill it. Your personal space can be the 5 inches around you in the subway, the 20 feet in front of and behind your car on the highway, or it can be your office, your computer workstation, even the sofa and coffee table in your living room at home. In our culture, people "own" their space, and they guard it with all the zealousness and high-minded principle of the U.S. Constitution and the Bill of Rights. What we do in our personal space is sacred.

That's why personal space "conflicts" can become so heated, and so, well, *personal*! As the owner of your space, you may feel entitled to perform any behavior you choose with impunity. Your neighbor or cohabitant, however, may disagree. Arguments over boundaries may ensue. It could get ugly. What rules do *you* apply to your sense of personal space? Do your rules agree with the rules of the people around you? Let's take a closer look.

Those Quirks Really Are Annoying

Sometimes, we just can't help it. Getting nervous? Twirl some hair or bite a nail. Concentrating? Jiggle that knee and tap that toe. Stressed-out? Clench that jaw. A lot of times your body will respond to whatever's going on in your mind by performing a behavior that gives you a physical release. We know someone who reduces mental stress by getting down on the floor and doing abdominal crunches. "It's healthy and centering," he says. Yeah, okay, but when you're in the middle of a brainstorming meeting it might be a little disconcerting to the 10 other participants.

And that's the point. The things we do to calm ourselves may be highly annoying and stress-provoking to others. Most of the time people don't even realize that what they're doing is annoying to other people until someone else points it out to them. Is that what's happened to you? If someone's told you that you do something with your body that drives them nuts, it's time to pull out your trusty Daily Habit Log and track the behavior until you begin to figure out how often you do it, where and when you do it, and who you'll actually do it in front of.

"It Wasn't Me": Owning Your Farts

Whoopi Goldberg (and where do you think she got her nickname?) has this to say about farting, "People have all kinds of techniques to avoid being found out. Some people keep pets around, so they can blame their farts on the cat, "Honey, cat farts bleach wood; they're so powerful." A lot of us pass gas, belch, crack our knuckles, shake our legs under the table (remember Diane Keaton in that scene from *Baby Boom*?), chew on our fingers, and snap gum, and we think other people aren't going to notice. We think we can slip it by just this once, without getting caught. As if, suddenly, we're invisible. And when we *do* get caught, it's "Who me?" Followed by a guilty, "And so what?"

You see, when you're in a public situation, you're a part of the whole big picture. What's going on isn't a movie that you're watching—you're a part of it. What you do, other people notice and have an opinion about. Making the transition in perception from passive viewer to active participant in the events of your life is the first step toward "owning" what you do, taking responsibility for *all* of your actions big and small, courageous *and* annoying. When you're uncomfortable or stressed, this can be a hard thing to do. For a moment, you lose the ability to see beyond yourself. In your *solipsism,* your panicky mind sends signals that make your body panicky and before you know it you're out of control: stomach rumbling, teeth clenched, and toe tapping a mile a minute.

The solution: Try a little stress management. If you can, excuse yourself from the situation and go somewhere private where you can behave however you'd like without embarrassing yourself or annoying others. At first, you might head straight for the nearest bathroom and compulsively indulge in your bad habit behavior. That's okay. After a minute or so though, take a deep breath, exhale. Do it again. Continue deep, focused breathing until you're calmer. The deep breathing allows your mind and body to work together constructively again—deep breaths signal the brain to release substances that soothe and relax the body, and sends more oxygen through the blood to the brain, increasing your ability to think and concentrate.

The important thing, though, is to own up to your reactions to stressful situations. Once you're more consciously aware of what you're doing—and you recognize what other people see and how they feel about it, you'll be able to gain the insights that'll help you change or control your behavior.

> **Strictly Speaking**
> **Solipsism** means total, blind self-absorption. It's the theory that only you exist, or can be proved to exist.

> **Cold Turkey**
> Look for other potentially bad habits that might exacerbate your body's strong need for physical release. If you're clenching your jaw, it might be worse if you're also drinking six cups of coffee a day. If you're a compulsive fidgeter, that cigarette may be too handy—and annoying—a prop.

"I Gotta Be Me": A Matter of Public Expression

Then there are those of us who know full well what we're doing and what affect it has on other people. It's called "pushing buttons." This passive-aggressive technique can psyche

217

other people out, make them angry, or plain just disgust them. But you can be sure of this, whatever their reactions, it's not going them make them love you more.

Strictly Speaking

Synergies are combinations of energy that produce something greater and more meaningful than the individual participants could create through their own energies. Positive synergies enhance and enrich our experience, while negative ones drain and hamper it.

Maybe you're someone who thinks belching is just a natural part of life and anyone who doesn't agree has been reading too much Miss Manners. You'd belch in the Secretary of State's direction at a White House dinner and be proud to be an American. After all, this is the land of free expression. But is this any way to win friends and influence people?

Or maybe your significant other is a little too compulsively neat for your taste, so you express your disapproval by drinking orange juice straight from the carton and leaving cherry lip balm stains all over the carton lip to mark your territory. This gets you into endless arguments about "letting you be you" but never addresses the real issue: That your partner's neatness is driving you nuts!

Or how about that guy who does abdominal crunches to center himself during meetings at work. Other coworkers may be more than just thrown off-guard by the oddness of it. They may be intimidated by an action that connotes a power play—I'm stronger than you are—relegating other participants to weaker roles in the discussion.

If what you're doing falls into this category, you'll want to reconsider whether your course of action really gets you anywhere. The point you're making by expressing yourself with such abandon doesn't involve an adult exchange of communication that respects viewpoints other than your own. Taking other people's thoughts and feelings into account creates a *synergy* that brings people together—instead of driving them apart.

Head to Toe Habits

So, how do you solve this problem of mind over matter? As we discovered earlier on in this book, a habit is one that your body/mind learns and comes to expect to perform. Breaking a habit you're so used to can seem as absurd as saying, "Now I'll stop brushing my teeth every day." You know that when you compulsively click through all the TV channels 12 times with the remote your roommates go ballistic, but that's the way you do it. How do you change?

Hair Twirling, Nose Picking, Teeth Grinding/Clenching, Gum Snapping, Knuckle Cracking, Nail Biting, Knee Shaking, Toe Tapping, Belching, Farting, and All Those Other Things You Do

Some physical *tics* and annoying behaviors are easier to remedy than others. You'll need to look at the following criteria.

➤ Does your bad habit tic cause you physical harm? For example, biting your nails until they bleed, clenching your jaw until you experience TMJ syndrome, holding in your personal releases because you're ultra-self-conscious—resulting in heartburn or gastrointestinal distress. If so, you'd be wise to discuss the problem with your primary care physician, who can help you come up with a treatment plan that allows you to break your bad habit and heal any damage done to your body.

A New Angle

About 20 percent of all Americans suffer from a condition called temporomandibular joint syndrome, also known as TMJ. In addition to clicking and popping and pain in the jaw, TMJ also includes symptoms of headache, neck pain, eye pain, tooth grinding, and ear aches. Dentists and doctors usually treat TMJ with medication, splints, and physical therapy exercises.

➤ Is your bad habit tic purely a physical response to stress in your environment, or a particularly stressful relationship? Try the deep breathing exercise we mentioned earlier in this chapter. If you can, remove yourself as quickly as possible from the stressful situation—take a walk outside to give yourself a chance to calm down and gain an objective perspective. Substituting your bad habit outlet with another less annoying or destructive behavior is another strategy. For example, instead of biting your nails, keep one of those hand massage balls that you squeeze to improve hand strength nearby and knead that whenever you feel the urge to bite.

Strictly Speaking

In psychological terms, a **tic** is defined as an involuntary, quick, repeated stereotypical movement or speech. Tics are expressions of emotional conflicts, or are caused by neurological conditions or as a side-effect of certain drugs.

One Day at a Time

Here's an easy way to recognize your urges to perform your bad habit tic and refocus your concentration in a new direction. Wear a rubber band around your wrist. Every time you get the urge, snap it. If you're snapping all day, you know your habit is out of control. But be careful, we don't want to turn you into a compulsive wrist-snapper!

➤ Like Ed Norton in *The Honeymooners*, do you use your physical tics to clear your head and gain perfectionist control over your environment? We all have things we need to do to enter that zone of full concentration. Maybe you need to prepare in a private place. Then, when it's your turn to give that piano solo or make that speech, just dive in and give yourself to the moment. You can't control everything!

➤ Are your physical tics and quirks directly aimed at making others in your life uncomfortable? If so, there may be deeper issues to address in your relationship than you're admitting to. If you lick a spoon and try to hang it on the tip of your nose every time your significant other wants to have a conversation about something serious, there's a bigger balance problem going on than your annoying behavior!

Stop It! Right Now!

Like any other bad habit, changing this one is going to take some time—and some understanding—from the people in your life. If all you're hearing is "You're doing it *again*!" ask for a little leeway and gentle reminders instead of constant nagging and hyper-vigilant attention to every little thing you're doing—or not doing! Remember, habits are *learned* behaviors. With some patience, you'll be able to retrain yourself into substitute behaviors that are more positive outlets for stress, or you'll be able to eliminate the need to perform your bad habit altogether by carefully addressing the relationship issues that caused you to act out in the first place.

You Can't Be Too Clean

If your habit involves excessive cleanliness of your physical person, you could be indulging in an obsessive-compulsive behavior. If you're a person who can't be too clean, perfectionism may be the too-high standard you hold in other areas of your life as well. And there may be issues in your past that have drawn you toward the need to control your environment.

Washing your hands until they become so dry they crack or bleed is not healthy—even if your scrupulous intention is to maintain good hygiene. Dermatologists agree that washing the skin too harshly or frequently isn't good for it. Being so afraid of germs that you become unable to function in an everyday environment, compulsively washing doorknobs or avoiding public places like the gym or the subway—ultimately holds you back from participating in and enjoying life day to day. Remember the character Anthony Edwards played on *Northern Exposure* before he became *E.R.*'s Dr. Green? He lived in a sanitized, germ-free eco-shelter, never leaving the house. But when Maggie coaxed him outside to "smell the roses," the guy adventured off on an exciting Greenpeace mission!

If your daily cleanliness rituals are overly elaborate, consider consulting your primary care physician or talking to a therapist about bringing your behavior back into a healthy perspective.

Can't We All Just Get Along?

Every year, the world fills up with more and more people and we find ourselves sharing our personal space not only with the people we love and the people we work with, but with strangers as well. It's important to acknowledge that we're part of a community, and that what we do has an affect on the people around us—the same way that what they do has an affect on us. In this stress-filled, fast-paced, twenty-first–century time, it's all too easy to develop physical strategies for releasing our stress and angst. If we recognize this, perhaps we can work together to develop habits that help us cope in mutually positive ways.

The Least You Need to Know

➤ Guarding your personal space—and asserting your right to behave as you please within it—are natural impulses.

➤ A lot of times you're not aware that your behavior is annoying until someone else points it out to you.

➤ Annoying tics and quirks are often just the body's way to release mental stress.

➤ Using tics and quirks to purposefully annoy others is passive-aggressive behavior.

➤ It's possible to trade in your annoying head-to-toe bad habits for positive behaviors that create good synergies with the people you encounter.

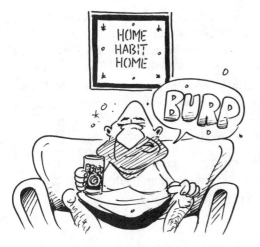

Home Is Where the Habit Is

Take a look around. Do the sheets on your bed have hospital corners, or does your bed closely resemble L.A. after an earthquake? Believe it or not, the way you treat your physical environment can reveal a lot about you—and how it can deeply affect your life and your relationships.

A little mess can go a long way, as can a little bit of organizing. You may be surprised to find that both messiness and neatness are really flip sides of the same coin: No matter how you toss it, it reveals a desire to control your environment and the other people who share it with you.

You Are What You Own

So, what's it like at your house? Too much stuff to even figure out what's there? Military discipline—rolled socks and shined shoes? Have friends and family compared you to Oscar Madison or Felix Unger just one too many times for you to be amused by it? Do you wonder why everyone makes wild excuses to avoid coming over?

You may be surprised when we tell you most housemates and houseguests feel equally uncomfortable in a room that's either too neat or too messy. That's because either style creates an intimidating environment for visitors. Don't believe us? Try this: Take a picture of each room in your house (this could also apply to your office at work...) and mount the pictures on a big sheet of white paper. Go out for a soothing cup of tea at a local cafe and take the montage of your house with you. Look at it. We mean really look at it. If you live alone, it's your self-portrait; a group portrait if you have roommates, or are a couple or a family. Is this a place you'd like to visit, much less live in?

The questions here, believe it or not, are the same ones physicists puzzle over on a grander scale: Is the universe based on order or chaos? And is there really any difference between the two? Let's take a look at what drives people to extremes.

Everything in Its Place

People don't become ridiculously organized overnight—it takes years and years of practice. Meticulous people believe they get great pleasure from knowing that everything has a place and can be found at a moment's notice. The pleasure of order gives the meticulous person the idea that the world makes sense—or can be made to make sense.... But this short-term pleasure may hold at bay what is often just a deep-seated fear of a dangerous world that they cannot manipulate, control, or tame—a place where anything can happen.

As a managing editor at a large publishing house, it's Laura's job to keep track of the scheduling and details of publication for 200 books each year—that's a lot of information to organize. Laura jokes that if she could get all that detail about the books out of her head, she'd have room to enjoy what's actually in the books. After all, it's a love of reading that led Laura to pursue a career in publishing in the first place. Laura has accidentally hit the compulsively ordered nail on the head. Like the Dutch boy with his finger in the dyke, Laura's too busy holding back chaos to enjoy much else.

The truth is, it's impossible to sustain order indefinitely. Isn't that a great law of science called the Second Law of Thermodynamics? Order inevitably tends toward disorder. Sooner or later, the unpredictable will happen.

Too Much Order

Clinically, the desire for order is a manifestation of the desire for control, and we all want to control our environment to some degree. When we try to control everything, though, desire has turned to compulsion—and it's time to examine underlying causes.

Some of the most controlling people we know ply their art insidiously, by making others believe that they're indispensable. This practice can run the gamut from the mother who still does her grown daughter's laundry every week because (she says) the daughter's so busy with her important job, to the father who's got the whole household running on a schedule—his schedule.

The Too Much Order Person (TMOP) will say things like, "If you'd put your keys in the same place every time you walked in, you wouldn't lose them," or "I don't know how you can find anything in this mess." The implication is that TMOP can find anything. Efficiency, the theory goes, makes TMOP indispensable; TMOP to the rescue!

TMOP's desire for order may also arise out of a need to control his or her immediate environment. There's so much uncertainty in the world today, the argument goes. Why, you can walk out your door and be run over by a truck! Maybe you can't control everything, but you can try to control your own space—and so you do.

What's Really Out of Place

The problem is that all this control is external. You're so busy putting a template on the world that you can conveniently avoid looking inside. And what's inside is a fear of the unknown. A life lived by rules and regulations—even ones that are self-imposed—takes away some of the responsibility and risk for making life's decisions, as well as the need to confront your own chaotic, unmanageable feelings, desires, and goals. Are you the person who is so disturbed by a painting that's hung crooked on the wall that you don't even see, much less appreciate what the artist has painted? Read on.

> ### A New Angle
>
> It's perfectly understandable why people today are afraid of things they can't control. This is partly because of our culture's rational belief system, where every effect has a cause, and every cause has an effect. Before the advent of modern science, though, people believed that events beyond their control were in the hands of the kings and queens, the gods, or the fates—and didn't worry so much about controlling the world themselves.

Which of the following statements are true about you?

➤ I become annoyed if my day goes off-schedule, so much so that I don't accomplish anything until the schedule goes back to where it should be.
*True*_____   *Not True*_____

➤ I appreciate a neat, clear desktop at work, but I'm not bothered by sitting in coworker's offices who can't even find the surface of their desks—that's their misfortune, not mine!   *True*_____   *Not True*_____

➤ During arguments my significant other will mess up all the bathroom towels and drop dirty clothes on the bathroom floor just to make me angrier—and it works!
*True*_____   *Not True*_____

One Day at a Time
Try writing down a list of adjectives in your Daily Habit Log that describes your actions throughout the day and how comfortable you felt in the places where you found yourself. Take a look at the list. Do these words describe you the way you'd like to be? The way you'd like others to see you? Are you efficient or adventurous? Clean or creative? Impatient or flexible?

➤ I like white rooms, or at least ones painted in solid colors. Patterns and, God forbid, plaids, make me nauseous. *True*_____   *Not True*_____

➤ I wash my eyeglasses four times a day with Windex and floss so often my dentist has told me to cut back. *True*_____   *Not True*_____

➤ I pick up after everyone: "Are you going to eat that banana?" "Can I rinse this coffee cup for you?" *True*_____   *Not True*_____

If you answered "true" to most of these questions, then you're paying far too much attention to adjusting the frame than you are to the beauty and adventure life paints as each day unfolds. If you're trying to dominate, regulate, manage, supervise, constrain (Hey, what are these synonyms for? Control!), you may want to learn to loosen up, let go, release, reveal…it's you, unchained!

Finding Your Inner Slob and Loving It!

Why not try something messy? Yes, you read it right. Start coloring outside the lines. You may feel a little uncomfortable at first, but it won't kill you.

Remember Laura, the managing editor? Well, Laura secretly wanted to do more than just read the books her company published—she wanted to write them. Problem: Laura gave all her energy, mental and physical, to organization. Also a perfectionist (as many compulsively neat people are), Laura realized she spent too many hours at the office making sure "everything got taken care of." What fell through the cracks was Laura herself; she neglected to take care of, to nurture, herself.

Is there something you've always been longing to do but the structure of your life just doesn't seem to allow it? We offer this challenge: Spend one hour each day doing something that has no boundaries, limits, or purpose other than to bring yourself joy. Paint, write, sing, garden. Remember to start small, spending just a few minutes on this new activity the first morning, and writing how it makes you feel in your Daily Habit Log. Pretty soon, you'll look forward to this time, expanding the length of time you spend and appreciating the sense of freedom it gives you.

And then find a place and a time in your life to be messy. Give the ones you love the same luxury. Maybe you own seven vacuum cleaners but you secretly yearn to pour dog treats on the carpet and watch the two dogs you love so much enjoy a treat-o-rama! Do it! Maybe your significant other wants to leave a pile of cookbooks out on the kitchen counter for the night; it's okay! Once you give yourself permission to dabble in one small mess, you may find a new freedom and flexibility in your approach to other areas of your life as well. Again, this is a process, and you may have to "work" at letting yourself go at the start.

The Chaos Theory

Of course, there are as many compulsive slobs as there are compulsive neatniks. We're not talking about a few dishes in the sink or a stack of newspapers next to the couch. We're talking about chaos.

In some cases, compulsive chaos can be attributed to Adult Attention Deficit Disorder (ADD), a condition that may result in an inability to focus one's attention on a particular task for more than a few minutes. Symptoms of ADD include a habitual inability to pay attention, excessive distractibility, difficulty with organization, impulsiveness, restlessness, and hyperactivity. If these symptoms make it hard for you to function on a daily basis, you should consider seeing a health care professional; ADD is highly treatable with medication and therapy.

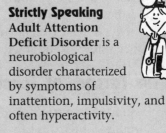

Strictly Speaking
Adult Attention Deficit Disorder is a neurobiological disorder characterized by symptoms of inattention, impulsivity, and often hyperactivity.

Most people's bad habit messiness, however, cannot be explained by an underlying neurobiological disorder, but instead is more likely to cover up a different kind of problem—the messy fear of giving up control. "Wait a minute," you say, "messiness doesn't mean control, it means out-of-control." Well, at first glance it might, but if you look a little deeper....

Compulsive sloppiness can take several forms. There's the executive who equates a messy desk with evidence of busy-ness, and who enjoys being the only one who can figure out what's going on. There's the packrat who starts by saving one magazine until, before he knows it, every room is stacked floor to ceiling. There's the young adult living away from home for the first time who's determined to prove that it doesn't matter if the dishes ever get washed.

By seemingly relinquishing control over their environments and situations, compulsive slobs are really manipulating and controlling the people and things in their lives through passive-aggressive behavior. Slobs believe they get pleasure from being disorganized, from the freedom of letting it all hang loose. But this short-term pleasure perhaps masks the same fear compulsively neat people have: the fear of a dangerous world that can't be manipulated, controlled, or tamed—a place where anything can happen. Both Felix Unger and Oscar Madison are afraid to risk taking responsibility for making life's decisions. Siddhartha (that's Buddha to you and me) said it best, "Pull the string too taut and it breaks; too loosely and it won't won't play." Either way, you're out of tune.

Damaging Disorder

Disorder starts out innocently enough. It starts with one sock on the floor, or one mail-order catalogue on the coffee table. Even when all the socks are on the floor, it's still possible to hunt for a pair, and, if you really have to pay a bill, you can paw through last month's mail (which you now find under as well as atop the coffee table) until you come across it. It's not like anything is lost, after all. You know it's in there somewhere.

The problem arises when the socks no longer hit the floor and the mail no longer hits the table—when everything just piles up wherever it falls, socks on the table, mail on the bed, dishes on top of the TV, and trash everywhere. When it gets to that point, you don't invite anyone over any more, and, if someone shows up, you joke that your maid's out sick this week. In other words, even *you* know there's a problem.

The Terrors of Tossing

Another side effect of compulsive chaos is the inability to throw anything away. In its milder forms, this can be a reluctance to toss an odd screw because you're sure enough it's just the size you'll need to fix the cabinet drawer. Full-blown, though, it means you can't throw out anything—not old *National Geographics*, because the kids might need them for school, or hopelessly snagged pantyhose, because, well, you know, you might need them for the clothes dryer vent. One friend of ours is absolutely unable to throw away a grocery bag, but instead neatly folds them and then crams them in the tiny space between the refrigerator and the wall. What she intends to do with them intrigues us all (and probably perplexes her as well).

In another rather sad case, a woman cleaning out her recently deceased mother-in-law's cupboards discovered the older woman had never, ever, thrown out a cottage cheese container: the stacks were a history of how Breakstone had changed their labels over the years. Not letting go, holding on to everything, is really a very controlled strategy to stop time. Remember the Dutch boy with his finger in the dyke?

> **Cold Turkey**
>
> If parting with all the stuff you've been hoarding in your house makes you break out in a cold sweat, relax! Experiment by asking some friends if you can store the last three years of Ad Age in their garage. If 30 days go by and you can't even remember that you ever subscribed to *Ad Age*, get your friends to toss them out!

Packrat alert: These days, recycling bins are everywhere. If you don't have home pick-up, even the smallest towns have drop-off points—or someone willing to pick up your paper, plastics, glass, and aluminum cans. And libraries now have back issues of hundreds of magazines available on microfiche or CD-ROM, so you don't even need to save those. Perhaps it will be easier to loosen your grip if you can imagine all that stuff going to good use somewhere else!

Creating Order

It's not so much a fear of what may be living in the back of the refrigerator as a fear of changing a habit that's grown as comfortable as an old shoe. And, just like a new pair of shoes, changing one's ways can hurt at first.

But those great old shoes were new once, too—and you didn't know how great they'd be until you'd worn them for awhile. And, just as you don't have to throw out the old shoes to break in a new pair, you don't have to clean up every area of your life to start on a new, less compulsive path.

The daunting problem in getting organized, though, is where to start. It's so daunting, in fact, many people never get past that step. So we'd like to make a simple suggestion: Start anywhere.

That's right. It doesn't matter if it's inside or out, upstairs or down, a room or a desk, you've just got to start somewhere. Let's start with your mail. Check the most appropriate action:

➤ **Two bills.**

Toss on the desk? ❑

Pay immediately? ❑

Put in your "financial box" where you keep your checkbook and other financial materials? ❑

➤ **Letter from Aunt Martha.**

Read immediately and toss on the desk? ❑

Read and place by your computer so you can write a reply after dinner? ❑

Throw it away (you never liked Aunt Martha, anyway)? ❑

➤ **Flyer from *Flyfishing Stories* saying they want you to resubscribe.**

Toss on the desk? ❑

Toss in the trash? ❑

Bill me later? ❑

➤ **This month's issue of *Blues Musician*.**

Toss in the trash?   ❏

Use it to level out that table that's been crooked for years?   ❏

Put it by the nightstand to read later?   ❏

➤ **Another clearinghouse sweepstakes—YOU'VE WON!!!**

Toss on the desk?   ❏

Toss in the trash?   ❏

Reply immediately (Eureka!)?   ❏

Getting organized means actually making decisions. Decisions that affect not only your environment, but your activities. Decisions that require opinions. How can you answer Aunt Martha's letter if you can't find it? And it you did find it, whatever would you say? Well, you won't know until you do it. (Could that be what you're really trying to express in the first place?)

Spend one hour a day going through something: a drawer, a shelf, a closet, a stack, anything. You may find that your efforts engage you with your environment, and with the other people in your life, in a new way—one that really does loosen you up more than it holds you in place.

Here are just a few more tips for building your organizational skills:

➤ Don't allow yourself to be overwhelmed by the "big picture." Tackle problems one by one, breaking each down into manageable pieces.

➤ Learn to be ruthless about obsolete paperwork or useless items. Throw them away or donate them to charity if appropriate.

➤ Use logic when designing space for your paperwork and personal belongings, but let your own unique personality shine through.

➤ Deal with each new item immediately. Sort mail within 24 hours and put away clothes as soon as they come out of the laundry, out of store packages, or off your body.

➤ Stop and think before you add new items to your home or work environment. Don't undermine the progress you've made by simply adding more stuff to the mix.

Heisenberg's Uncertainty Principle

Whose uncertainty what? We're back to the habits of the universe. According to Heisenberg's Uncertainty Principle nothing in the universe can be pinned down. Every particle is always in motion. By the time you give it a location, it's already moved. So we can't stop time and we can't stop matter. The dance of order and chaos continues un-abated, and neither succeeds at gaining control. The best we humans can do is join in the process, the act of living, a day at a time, knowing that only one thing is certain in life: Nothing is certain! That said, it's important that you take the time to recognize and reward yourself for every bit of success you achieve in breaking your organizational bad habits. You're learning to go with the flow!

The Least You Need to Know

➤ The desire for too much order or too much disorder is a manifestation of a need to control your environment.

➤ You can "allow" yourself to be messy or neat in one area of your life.

➤ Compulsive neatness or sloppiness can mask a fear of change.

➤ You, too, can learn to go with the flow.

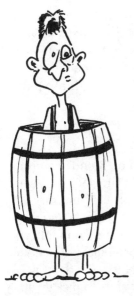

Finally, Fiscal Fidelity

Rich people exist. We know it 'cause we've seen them on TV, read about them in magazines, maybe even know a few of them. But chances are, if your bad habits fall into the realm of the almighty dollar, you aren't one of them. That's not to say, of course, that if you could only stop spending money like it's water and start sticking to a realistic budget, you too might just be hobnobbing with Donald Trump—or at least be able to afford to pay your mortgage on time every month! One thing's for sure: Until you learn how to control your financial life, it'll certainly control you.

Your Money Style

Without question, there are as many different money styles as snowflakes and fingerprints. Some people are inveterate savers, who derive pleasure from seeing money accrue in bank accounts, while others have a more carefree attitude that allows them to spend more freely—but within certain limits. Both types can manage quite well, as long as they avoid a few of the most common money traps. These include: over-spending, disorganized financial records, tax trouble, and budget phobia. We'll explain these common woes to you in this chapter, as well as give you some tips to start getting you out of the money pit. And later, we'll have advice for you "pie-in-the-sky types" who think all the money in the world is right around the corner.

Spending Too Much?

"This week, I swear I won't waste any money," you vow to yourself on Monday morning. But on the way to work, you just have to have that double hazelnut latte ($3.50). Then the muffin cart comes around, and, well, who can resist the chocolate chip muffins ($1.50). Your coworkers suggest sushi for lunch, and you can't resist ($6.60, with tip). During an afternoon lull, you flip through a catalogue and see some fabulous shoes. You casually dial the toll-free number ($49.95). On the way home, you stop by the local discount store to pick up a few necessities, and come out with a new portable CD player, ten new CDs (there was a great sale…), and a handy carrying case, plus the toilet paper and detergent you really needed ($259.99). After picking up a pizza on the way home, you realize you've spent more than $300 dollars in just under 12 hours. It's so easy to spend money in America today! The opportunities bombard us at every turn. On the Internet, on television, the radio, and around every corner, great bargains, super savings, and "the product of your dreams" await. So why are some of us able to turn a blind eye to all this temptation, while others keep their money in continuous motion from paycheck deposit to ATM withdrawal? The answer: Habit!

Cold Turkey
Loans by banks, credit card companies, even the government, are serious money-making opportunities—for the LENDER, not the borrower. If you apply for a loan, make sure you get the figures: the loan amount versus what you'll pay making the minimum payments over the life of the loan. (Remember interest?) Yikes! Ask yourself if you can possibly pay cash, do without, or do with less.

Some people have trouble with overspending because of stress related directly to money. But other people find their overspending habit is triggered by any number of other emotional and practical challenges. In some cases, this can result in a full-fledged addiction. If you think your spending habits might be a bigger problem, answer these questions:

1. Do you habitually take off for the stores when you've experienced a set-back or disappointment? *Yes____ No____*

2. Are your spending habits emotionally disturbing to you, or do they create chaos in your life? *Yes____ No____*

3. Do your shopping habits create conflicts with someone close to you?
   *Yes*____ *No*____

4. As a general rule, when you shop do you feel a rush of euphoria mixed with feelings of anxiety? *Yes*____ *No*____

5. When you return home after shopping, do you feel guilty, ashamed, embarrassed, or confused? *Yes*____ *No*____

If you answer "yes" to even one or two of these questions, your bad habit may be becoming a problem that requires intervention from a health professional. Even if you aren't a compulsive shopper, however, you still may need to retrain yourself to understand the difference between "need" and "want." Could it be that the designer suit you crave is really a substitute for companionship or intellectual stimulation or just a break from the boredom you feel on a Saturday afternoon? Once you identify the reasons you overspend, and learn to think long and hard about shelling out a single dime for anything that isn't truly in the "need" category, you'll start to gain financial control. Here are some tips to get you started:

➤ **Out of sight, out of mind.** If you haven't yet purchased the latest gazillion megahertz, gigabyte computer that does everything but make breakfast, walk away and make do with your perfectly serviceable, two-year-old workhorse. Not knowing what you're missing isn't always such a bad thing.

➤ **Keep track.** Here we go again with the Daily Habit Log. Only this time, you'll be tracking every single dime you spend (at least for awhile). Buy that hazelnut latte, write down what it costs you. Every day. At the end of each week, tally up your totals. You'll be shocked and appalled at first, but it'll help you cut back.

➤ **Eat in.** Learn to cook. It's fun, and it saves tons of money compared to restaurant or take-out costs. Besides, it's "in" to be a homebody these days. Just ask the rich and famous Martha Stewart!

➤ **Take it with you.** Brew your own gourmet coffee at home and bring it to work in a thermos. Brown-bag your lunch. Many of us spend insane amounts on food and drink throughout the day at work.

➤ **Buy close to home.** We know how much fun it is to shop from the living room couch. But unless it's an amazing deal, avoid buying from catalogues and TV shopping networks. By the time you add shipping and handling charges and pay for all the returns of clothes that don't fit because you don't have the same body as the model, you'll have spent far more than you would've in a day shopping the sales at the outlet mall.

Cold Turkey
Look before you leap! Impulse buying is the bane of your healthy bank account. Before you buy anything, ask yourself four questions: Do I need it? Do I have to have it right now? What will happen if I don't buy it? How have I managed this long without it?

➤ **Don't join the "clubs."** Watch out for other mail-order traps like book and CD clubs. Sure, you get lots of free stuff up front, but after that, you've usually got to buy a large number of very over-priced products, especially when you add the inflated shipping charges. It isn't worth it.

➤ **Quit smoking.** In addition to destroying your health, smoking is a very expensive habit. (See Chapter 12 if you need more convincing!)

➤ **Treat yourself well.** You'll only be setting yourself up for a fall if you set too strict a limit on your spending; you're likely to indulge in a dangerous shopping "binge." Make room in your budget for occasional splurges—just don't go overboard.

Financial Records in Disarray?

You don't spend that much money—at least, you don't think you do. On the other hand, you'd have no way of knowing because you haven't balanced your checkbook in six years. Bank statements usually land, unopened, in the trash. And when you bounce a check, you're always afraid to open the envelope revealing the awful truth. You pray the recipient of your bogus check sends it back through and that the money really is there this time to cover it.

Shoddy record-keeping is another bad habit, and one that can get you into a heap of financial trouble. One bounced check usually costs you a fee from your bank and a fee from the bouncee. Plus, if you've got no idea where your money goes, you're much more likely to waste it. Wouldn't you rather have a little financial security and a lot less financial stress?

People who have trouble organizing their financial records tend to experience high levels of stress about money, simply because they don't know whether they have it or not. (If you're filthy rich and just can't be bothered to balance your checkbook, that's another matter. You can hire someone to do it!)

The good news: You can set yourself free from money anxiety by applying a little structure and organization to your finances—even if what you find out is that you don't have as much money as you thought. At least you'll know the truth, and can spend accordingly, even start getting a little ahead.

To get started on your way to financial freedom, start fresh. Don't write any checks until all outstanding checks have been paid out—usually about one week after you've written your last check. Then call your bank to find out your balance and write it down. NEVER, EVER write a check or make an ATM withdrawal without recording it and subtracting it from the total balance. To make things even easier, invest in a good financial software program (e.g., Quicken or Microsoft Money), which can help you balance your checkbook, illustrate how you allocate your money in graph form, and even help you create a budget.

Tax Nightmares?

Uh-oh, the IRS! Perhaps someday, the government will finally simplify the tax code and make life easier for virtually everyone in the United States. Until that day, however, complicated tax forms are a necessary evil all Americans encounter.

Tax laws change almost as often as hem lines, which makes it especially tough for the financially challenged. What's deductible, what's not, and what goes where are just a few of the questions you face every year. What's a person to do?

Hire an accountant. For about $300 (maybe much less), a competent, knowledgeable person, who actually *chooses* to deal with the IRS, will prepare your returns for you. You'll almost definitely want to hire an accountant if you're self-employed, have employees, or have any other unusual tax situation, unless you're very ambitious and love to figure out these things on your own (in which case, we doubt you need to be reading this chapter). Accountants are a great investment of your money, especially since their tax-related fees are tax-deductible!

If you decide to knuckle down and do your taxes yourself, allow yourself plenty of time to organize your records, find answers to your questions, and double-check your figures. (If you have trouble with procrastination, read Chapter 17 first!) Fortunately, there're lots of good books, computer programs, and telephone help lines to aid you in your quest for tax security.

Experiencing Budget Phobia?

"But I don't want to balance my assets against my expenditures, or whatever it is a budget's supposed to do! I just want to spend!" you wail. If so, you're not alone. Budget phobia is really pretty common, even though making a budget and sticking to it leads to sanity and, often, a pretty healthy savings account after awhile! Indeed, budgets can be lifesavers, especially for people who tend to overspend without realizing it or who have trouble maintaining accurate financial records.

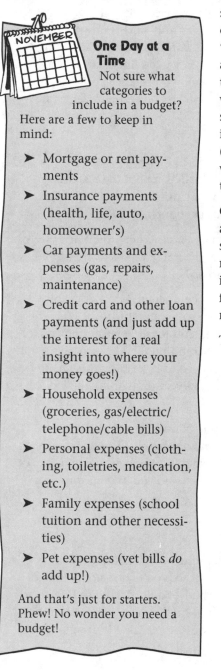

One Day at a Time

Not sure what categories to include in a budget? Here are a few to keep in mind:

➤ Mortgage or rent payments

➤ Insurance payments (health, life, auto, homeowner's)

➤ Car payments and expenses (gas, repairs, maintenance)

➤ Credit card and other loan payments (and just add up the interest for a real insight into where your money goes!)

➤ Household expenses (groceries, gas/electric/telephone/cable bills)

➤ Personal expenses (clothing, toiletries, medication, etc.)

➤ Family expenses (school tuition and other necessities)

➤ Pet expenses (vet bills *do* add up!)

And that's just for starters. Phew! No wonder you need a budget!

Does using the word "choice" in relation to "budget" seem strange to you? If so, you've discovered your biggest obstacle to financial freedom. "Budget" doesn't mean "restriction" or "denial." Budget means "choice." Creating a budget means making decisions about what's important to you, now and in the future. You set your goals and then, work within the parameter of your financial assets (your salary, your set expenses). You may need to limit spending in certain areas (which you choose) to meet those goals (which you've chosen). In the end, the positive outcome will outweigh the limitations because you've set the agenda to begin with. You choose.

Of course, sometimes non-budgeted expenses arise, such as an unexpected breakdown of your central air-conditioning system in August or an unplanned trip to the emergency room when Junior decides to play Spiderman by shimmying up the rain gutter. But that's what savings accounts are for, and we all know you'll never get around to putting money into that savings account unless you keep a budget.

Try these three easy steps to a working budget:

➤ **Universal understanding.** If you're not in this alone—if you've got a spouse, children, and/or dependent parents—it's essential that everyone understand (if not necessarily agree on) the family's financial goals and priorities.

➤ **Track your assets and expenditures.** Yes, again. Break out that Daily Habit Log and write down every cent you spend and every cent you earn. Compare the log to your budget and find out where your money goes.

➤ **Cut out the fat.** Keep chipping away at the non-essentials until your expenses equal your income. Don't forget to allot some money each month for savings—most advisors recommend at least 10 percent of your income—and for unexpected expenses.

The Thrill of a Gamble

Call it the lazy person's American dream: Something for (almost) nothing. You'd be crazy not to get excited about the prospect of huge sums of money dropped in your lap just because you purchased a lottery ticket for a dollar or stuck a few quarters in a slot machine. But the truth is, there's no such thing as a free lunch. Whether your preference is Vegas or bingo, lottery tickets or poker with your buddies, the thrill you derive from a gamble often costs far more than it's worth.

From the Casino to the Stock Market

You don't need a blackjack table to be a gambler. You can get your thrill by betting on horse races or sports events like the Super Bowl, buying lottery tickets, playing bingo, gambling on the Internet, or investing in the stock market. You might even bet for the heck of it: "I'll bet you 20 bucks you can't throw that peanut up in the air and catch it in your mouth on the first try!" "Oh yeah? I'll bet I can, and I'll bet you $100 I can do it 10 times in a row!"

There's certainly nothing wrong with living on the edge every once in awhile—if you can afford it. And the stock market is now considered a fairly sound investment if handled wisely. However, when gambling becomes a habit you can't support, financially or emotionally, you've got a problem. And you're not alone. According to recent studies, five percent of adults and eight percent of teens display compulsive gambling tendencies, and in its first year of operation alone, the Gambling Help Line received over 100,000 calls from troubled gamblers and their families.

"I Know When to Stop..."

Lots of people gamble for fun and know when to stop. But if you have trouble pulling back those reins, you may be heading toward the line that separates people who gamble for entertainment from people who gamble compulsively. Ask yourself the following 20 questions, provided by Gamblers Anonymous, to determine whether you might have a problem with compulsive gambling:

1. Did you ever lose time from work or school due to gambling?
   Yes____ No____

2. Has gambling ever made your home life unhappy?   Yes____ No____

3. Did gambling affect your reputation?   Yes____ No____

4. Have you ever felt remorse after gambling?   Yes____ No____

5. Did you ever gamble to get money with which to pay debts or otherwise solve financial difficulties?   Yes____ No____

6. Did gambling cause a decrease in your ambition or efficiency?
   *Yes*____ *No*____

7. After losing did you feel you must return as soon as possible and win back your losses? *Yes*____ *No*____

8. After a win did you have a strong urge to return and win more? *Yes*____ *No*____

9. Did you often gamble until your last dollar was gone? *Yes*____ *No*____

10. Did you ever borrow to finance your gambling? *Yes*____ *No*____

11. Have you ever sold anything to finance gambling? *Yes*____ *No*____

12. Were you reluctant to use "gambling money" for normal expenditures?
    *Yes*____ *No*____

13. Did gambling make you careless of the welfare of your family?
    *Yes*____ *No*____

14. Did you ever gamble longer than you had planned? *Yes*____ *No*____

15. Have you ever gambled to escape worry or trouble? *Yes*____ *No*____

16. Have you ever committed, or considered committing, an illegal act to finance gambling? *Yes*____ *No*____

17. Did gambling cause you to have difficulty sleeping? *Yes*____ *No*____

18. Do arguments, disappointments, or frustrations create within you an urge to gamble? *Yes*____ *No*____

19. Did you ever have an urge to celebrate any good fortune by a few hours of gambling? *Yes*____ *No*____

20. Have you ever considered self destruction as a result of your gambling?
    *Yes*____ *No*____

Most compulsive gamblers will answer "yes" to at least seven of these questions. If this sounds like you, please seek professional help. There are plenty of people out there, just like you, who can help you break this bad habit before it breaks you.

Playing It Safe

Everyone likes a little excitement in their lives once in awhile, but when it comes to your money, unless you've got loads to throw around, you're better off playing it safe. Take other sorts of risks: Ask out that beautiful person. Register for a college class, even though you're pushing 50. Take a trip somewhere you've never been before, even though there are no relatives to visit and no business to conduct. Say, "I love you," to your teenage child. Join that fitness club and dare to get really buff. The point is, life can be full of excitement and risks that don't have to compromise your financial integrity or cause large, scary-looking thugs to come knocking on your door to collect. Redirect your thrill-seeking to more productive outlets and you won't even miss that boring old casino.

Ralph Kramdenitis: Another Get-Rich-Quick Scheme

One last risk to your financial freedom, and it's directly related to the "Something for Nothing" delusion. It's the "Get Rich Quick" delusion. You've heard the saying: If it sounds too good to be true, it probably is. Well, you're hearing it again. (And if you haven't heard it, Ralph Kramden's got some shares in the Brooklyn Bridge that have your name all over them!)

Whether it's a *pyramid scheme*, a chain letter, "magic" diet pills, long-distance service, or real estate investment, remember that nobody makes money without effort. The people who do make a killing at any of these are few indeed, and worked much harder than they let on. For the rest of us, dreaming of something we can do in our spare time (meaning the approximately three minutes of spare time we have per day) that will make us millionaires seems like a dream come true. But after you've invested your money and lost it, you're going to wake up and realize it really was more like a nightmare.

> **Strictly Speaking**
> Pyramid, or Ponzi, schemes are illegal and fraudulent. Recruits "invest" money with recruiters and then enlist new recruits to "invest." Only the people at the very top of the pyramid make any money—the rest usually lose, big time. Recruiting people to participate in a pyramid scheme is a felony in many states.

When it comes to your money, invest it wisely, cautiously, and frugally. If you're really searching for independence and the chance to be an entrepreneur, do lots of research and then invest your money in starting your own business. In the meantime, don't let shysters and con artists rob you of your hard-earned cash. Be smart and sensible. Listen to your common sense. And NEVER give out financial information to someone who calls to solicit you over the telephone for ANY reason—keep your credit card account numbers, bank account numbers, social security number, and other financial data private. You never know who's *really* on the other end of the line.

A New Angle

To illustrate why pyramid schemes are unworkable, *The Skeptic's Dictionary* says, "If a pyramid were started by a human being at the top with just 10 people beneath him, and 100 beneath them, and 1,000 beneath them, etc., the pyramid would involve everyone on earth in just 10 layers of people with "one con man on top."

Putting Your Financial House in Order

Now that you've found out how to stop overspending, start organizing, stick to a budget, quench your urge to gamble your money away, and just say no to get-rich-quick schemes, how do you actually start practicing fiscal fidelity? Try these tips:

➤ **Stop charging.** Don't get any more credit cards. Pay off the ones you have, then keep the balances low enough that you can pay them off each month. Not that much control? Then cut up the cards you have and throw them away. Pay cash. Old fashioned, maybe, but it works, and it helps you live within your means!

➤ **Spend down your debts.** Add just $50 dollars a month to your minimum credit card payment, and you'll drastically reduce the interest you'll pay and the time you'll spend paying off the balance.

➤ **Live within your means.** You cannot have the Ferrari!

➤ **Start saving, even if it hurts.** Because, like all good habits, the end result is far better than any interim inconvenience. Check with your employee benefits department: Many companies have 401K savings plans that involve placing a set amount of money from each paycheck, into a savings account—a relatively painless way to "pay yourself first."

➤ **Learn to do-it-yourself.** Cook your own meals, learn how to fix your car or appliances when they break down, start a baby-sitting co-op, practice preventive medicine by keeping yourself healthy, make your own gifts, and research the opportunities for free entertainment in your area—from nature parks to free movies at the library. You never know, you just might have some fun along the way.

The Least You Need to Know

➤ Overspending, disorganized financial records, tax problems, and fear of a budget all contribute to a serious financial bad habit.

➤ If you think you have a gambling problem, you probably do. Consider seeking professional help.

➤ Get-rich-quick schemes more often yield net losses than net gains.

➤ Life can be full of thrills and excitement that don't risk your financial integrity—the best things in life really *are* free!

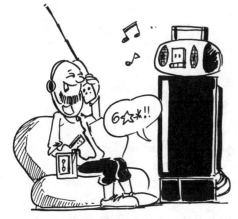

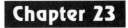

Chapter 23

Loving an Electronic High

In This Chapter

➤ The impact of electronic media

➤ Identifying your electronic habits

➤ The false intimacy of virtual reality

➤ Making time for the here and now

There's a great scene at the beginning of the movie *Throw Momma from the Train*. Billy Crystal plays a writer who sits before a blank sheet of paper in his typewriter (it was the pre-PC '80s...) and stares. Then he types an opening sentence, reads it, hates it, tears it up. Tries again. Tears it up. Stares some more. Cleans his desk. Sharpens some pencils. Gets some coffee. Stares some more.

And then he sees it.

The TV remote control. It appears before him like an angel of mercy. He goes for it, presses the magic button, the TV screen lights up, and the work never gets done. Not that day at least.

Sound familiar to you? In this Information Age many of us feel overworked, overbooked, overwhelmed, and just plain too tired (we think) to give that extra ounce of effort to complicated relationships and activities, and the electronic media easily seduces us with the offer of a perfect escape. It requires no commitment, little energy, and it's always, always there, ready to distract and amuse us.

Do you use the easy escape of the television or computer to avoid dealing with a difficult task or relationship? Have you come to depend on television shows or Internet surfing to be your companions, your intimate partners? Or maybe it's the telephone, cell phone, and fax that takes up your time, distracting you from the here and now with their false sense of urgency and connection?

Tuning In, Tuning Out

If you fall victim to the many temptations offered by the electronic media, you're among friends here. According to recent surveys, almost half of the Americans say they watch too much TV—and they're only the ones who admit it. So many people acknowledge that their use of the Internet is out of control that psychologists have now named the problem Internet Addiction Disorder, or IAD. And by observation alone, you can tell that telephone use has gotten completely out of hand: People at restaurant tables, surrounded by friends, but with a cell phone attached to their ear; or driving down a beautiful country road with a chance to observe nature along the way, but instead chatting non-stop on the car phone.

What's going on? How did these communication tools become such insidious escape hatches from the important pursuit of human connections? How can you find your way back from virtual reality to *real* reality?

The Boob Tube Personified

Do you think you might have trouble controlling how much television you watch? Answer these questions to see how bad it's gotten:

1. What's the first thing you do when you get home from work?

    (a) Kiss your spouse or significant other.

    (b) Play with the dog.

    (c) Turn on the television.

2. On a free Friday night, you'd prefer to:

    (a) Play a game of pick-up basketball.

    (b) Flip through an issue of *Sports Illustrated*.

    (c) Watch a game on TV while flipping between the game and *Millenium*?

246

3. You watch television for:

   (a) An hour or two of amusement.

   (b) Sixty minutes of news and information.

   (c) Endless mind-numbing distraction.

4. When you turn off the TV, you feel:

   (a) Relaxed.

   (b) Stimulated.

   (c) It turns off?!

5. Your remote control is:

   (a) A handy tool.

   (b) Hasn't been seen for a few days.

   (c) Your best friend in the whole wide world.

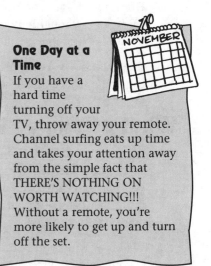

One Day at a Time

If you have a hard time turning off your TV, throw away your remote. Channel surfing eats up time and takes your attention away from the simple fact that THERE'S NOTHING ON WORTH WATCHING!!! Without a remote, you're more likely to get up and turn off the set.

How did you do? Too many "C" answers? Well, read on to see just how insidious watching television can be.

"Not unlike drugs or alcohol, the television experience allows the participant to blot out the real world and enter into a pleasurable and passive mental state," wrote Marie Winn, the author of the 1977 bestseller, *The Plug-In Drug*. "The worries and anxiety of reality are effectively deferred by becoming absorbed in a television program...." What could be a more perfect release than television and the "people" who populate it, people with seemingly more compelling problems than your own, but who can solve them in 30 or 60 minutes of distracting drama or comedy?

We know what you're thinking. "Sure, I like to watch television. Who doesn't? But I'm not obsessive. I can turn it off any time I want." Are you sure? Twenty years ago Marie Winn made another statement that still rings true: "People overestimate their control over television watching.... With television pleasures available, those other experiences (reading, conversing, practicing hobbies) seem less attractive, more difficult somehow." And that was before cable and video!

Think of it this way: 66 percent of American homes have three or more television sets. The number of hours per day the TV is on is 6 hours and 47 minutes (eight hours at work, eight hours asleep—that leaves two hours for all other activities!). A startling 66 percent of Americans watch TV while eating dinner (that sure cuts down on family conversation, doesn't it?). Fifty-four percent of American children have a TV in their bedrooms.

(Whatever happened to playing checkers with friends or reading comic books and Nancy Drew?) And—are you sitting down?—the average American youth watches 1,500 hours of TV in a year, roughly twice as much time as they spend in school. Need we say more? Most of us watch too much TV.

The good news: You CAN learn to say no to the boob tube. The first step: Wanting to. At the end of this chapter, you'll find out ways to break free from the airwaves.

What a Tangled Web You Weave

It's easier to sit back and let things happen, isn't it? To forego decision-making, turn off your brain, and just point and click. Easier, perhaps, but in the end, not very valuable, as you may have discovered if you've spent too much time surfing the Net. In the end, this is another passive activity, one that doesn't require you to become intellectually and emotionally engaged.

We know what you're thinking: It's only geeky, pimply, overweight teenage boys who become addicted to computers and the *Internet*. Not you. You've got a career, children, pets—you're not spending much time with them because of the computer, but you've got them.

Well, cast aside your assumptions. If you think you're spending more time than you should playing computer games, surfing the Web, or "chatting" with strangers, you probably are. And you're not alone. Although researchers can't put a number on how many Internet-addicted people are out there, they do know that the population ranges in age from 14 to 74 and includes a wide variety of personality types.

Strictly Speaking
The **Internet** is a network of information —social, financial, and general interest— that's transmitted electronically over telephone cables through modems into computers. As of January 1997, approximately 57 million people worldwide use the Internet.

What's the attraction of the computer and the Net? There are plenty of them. Look at the people you can be, with just a computer, a modem, and a telephone line:

The Pretender. Are you on the shy side? Do you have trouble talking to members of the opposite sex? Do you feel insecure about your looks? If so, you might be attracted to Internet chat rooms. A chat room can be nothing more than an enormous masquerade ball, where you can put on any costume—transforming yourself into any type of person you can imagine—and never have to take it off. You can hide your appearance, assume alternate personas and genders, and feel far less inhibited than you might be in face-to-face interactions.

People who have difficulty with communicating face to face, for any reason, are the ones most likely to become dependent on electronic forms of communication, particularly the

Internet. They're looking for ways to achieve anonymous "intimacy"—the illusion of social relationships that are free of awkwardness, discomfort, and fear of rejection. Although participating in chat rooms and calling 900 phone numbers may help raise self-esteem and self-confidence in the short term—and in rare instances can lead to the formation of real-life friendships and romances—in the end, you may very well end up alone, in the dark, staring at a blinking screen or holding the phone receiver in one hand and the TV remote in the other.

The Media Awed. Another breed of Net addicts lose themselves in the colorful, information-packed Web. They sign on thinking they'll look up that one article about the new TV line-up (talk about a tangled web!), and end up surfing through hyperlink after hyperlink, ending up reading about a resort in Thailand. Yes, we agree, the Internet is a stimulating educational tool, but so is the library; so are the books that line your shelves; the magazines on your coffee table (Did we say coffee?); and conversation with friends, family, and colleagues at work. Use the Internet for all of the wonderful information it can provide you, but be careful not to let it become a substitute for real-life interaction.

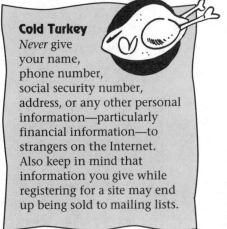

Cold Turkey
Never give your name, phone number, social security number, address, or any other personal information—particularly financial information—to strangers on the Internet. Also keep in mind that information you give while registering for a site may end up being sold to mailing lists.

The Gamester. Have a rough day at work? Angry at the kids for not cleaning their rooms? Tired of fighting a losing battle for respect from your parents or your spouse? Then play a computer game and outwit them—or even pretend to blow them all to smithereens. Want to take a "little break" from a writing task? Slide your mouse up to the Solitaire icon and you're on your way. If you can limit yourself to one or two games, you can relieve some stress and have some fun. But if the next time you look up from the screen is three hours later, you've done nothing to solve your problems except redden your eyes and tire your brain.

Do any of these profiles fit you? All of them? Here's a quiz that might help further identify and determine the extent of your Internet habit:

1. Do you spend more time than you think is appropriate surfing the Net? *Yes*____ *No*____

2. Do you have difficulty limiting your time online? *Yes*____ *No*____

3. Have any of your friends or family members complained about the time you spend at your computer? *Yes*____ *No*____

4. Do you find it hard to stay away from the Net for several days at a time? *Yes*____ *No*____

5. Has either your work or your personal life suffered as a result of your time on the Net? *Yes*____ *No*____

6. Have you tried unsuccessfully to curtail your use of the Net? *Yes*____ *No*____

7. Do you derive much of your pleasure and satisfaction in life from being on the Net? *Yes*____ *No*____

8. Have you stopped enjoying other once pleasurable hobbies or activities to make time for your Net activities? *Yes*____ *No*__

If you've answered "yes" to just one or two questions, your Internet habits are in pretty good shape. Let's face it: The Internet is an integral and fascinating part of the world, and it makes sense to play with it.

If you've answered "yes" to three to five questions, you might be heading for a problem. You're probably spending more time than you can afford exploring the Web or in chat rooms, which means you're probably neglecting your relationships, work, or other leisure activities.

If you've answered "yes" to more than five or six questions, you've got to start getting your Internet use under control. It's begun to take over your life, preventing you from facing important issues, establishing and maintaining important relationships, and having a life away from an inanimate, impersonal screen. We'll show you how just a little later.

A New Angle

In 1997, Senator Lauch Faircloth, Republican from North Carolina, became so incensed when he saw members of his staff playing games on the office PCs that he responded by proposing legislation. The measure would require federal agencies to remove any games currently installed on their computers, and prohibit the purchase of new machines with pre-loaded games.

Here a Phone, There a Phone

In the United States alone, there are now nearly 200 million telephones, not counting the increasingly ubiquitous cell phones. (Just try to imagine the noise that would erupt if even half of them rang at the same time. Why half? The other half would be the ones calling of course!) The telephone is without doubt an essential piece of equipment now that the world has become so large, so complicated, and so interdependent.

But there's a limit. If you can't count the number of phone calls you take or make during the course of day, if you use the phone as an excuse not to leave the house or give your full attention to another task, you may have a problem, one that requires a little of the old "breaking bad habits" magic!

Breaking Free from the Airwaves

Dealing with Internet, television, and telephone bad habits is no different than dealing with any other bad habit. You first have to gain an understanding of what role the habit plays in your life.

➤ **Avoidance.** You probably know by now that by turning your attention away from what is stressful but important, and toward something mindless like a TV show or Internet chat room, you're never going to make progress or resolve problem situations. Refocus your attention and you'll feel much better about yourself and about your chances of meeting your goals.

➤ **Boredom.** Trust us when we say this: Endless TV watching, Internet surfing, or telephone talking will not actually amuse or stimulate you. Instead, you'll end up feeling drained, lazy, unworthy, and, believe it or not, even more bored. To relieve boredom, you need to become involved in something that engages you in an active, not a passive way.

➤ **Loneliness.** Loneliness is probably the most common and devastating chronic illness in the United States. And, on the surface, what could be a better cure than thousands of "people"—characters in TV shows or Internet chatters—entering your living room in the flick of a switch? What's that phone ad: Reach out and touch someone? If only Americans went out and did that a little bit more!

Breakthroughs in the speed and ease of communication are making the times we live in as exciting as the Renaissance in the fifteenth century when the *Guttenberg Bible* rolled off the first printing press and books changed the world. No doubt, television, telephones, faxes, e-mails, and the Internet represent a major advancement in human potential—up there with Neil Armstrong's first footprint on the moon. But we need to use these communication tools in a way that doesn't paradoxically alienate us from the face-to-face contact that makes us uniquely human. If we try to live only in our minds, we're losing touch with our bodies, with other people in our community, and with the world around us.

There are several techniques you can learn that will help you avoid bad electronic habits. Here are a few to get you started:

251

➤ **Maintain your Daily Habit Log.** We're not nagging, honest we're not. But until you understand what it is you're trying to avoid by flicking that electronic switch or dialing that phone, you won't be able to stop yourself from doing it. Every time you feel the urge to tune in, write it down. Explore your feelings before, during, and after.

➤ **Schedule alternate activities.** The really seductive part about TVs, computers, and phones is that they're right there in front of you, ready and willing to take you away. If you've planned specific activities ahead of time—tickets to a game, a dinner date with friends, sessions with a personal trainer—you'll be far less likely to stay home and veg out.

➤ **Set and maintain a strict time limit for electronic activities.** Can't live without CNN? Terrific. Watch for one hour, then make yourself get up and do something else—even if it's for 15 minutes, which is usually enough to break the "human-TV connection" that otherwise seems iron-clad. Want to play an interactive computer game? Fabulous. Just log off as soon as that one game is over—win or lose.

➤ **Unplug—the phone, the computer, the television—for several hours during the day.** Phones have answering machines, computers store e-mail, and VCRs tape "must-see TV" for you to retrieve and enjoy later. During your time-out, read a book, make love, take a long walk around the neighborhood, learn to knit. Have fun.

A New Angle

Every year, an organization called TV-Free America sponsors a TV-Turnoff Week during which families are encouraged to turn off the television and find other activities to occupy their time—for an entire week. During the 1996 TV-Turnoff Week, organizers estimated that more than a million people stopped watching the tube. In fact, TV-Free America received more than 10,000 personal letters from kids and adults raving about their week without TV. Why don't you try it this year?

➤ **Start a new venture.** While activities like dinners out and exercise sessions will help distract you, the best way to break your electronic bad habit is to develop a true and abiding passion for something else: Think of what you could do with the hours you watch TV or surf the Net every night. Get a graduate degree? Learn a new language? Finish the basement guest room? The possibilities are limitless.

➤ **Eat all your meals away from the television, computer, and telephone.** The best time to communicate with your loved ones is at the table as you share food, conversation, and laughter. Not only will you be less likely to find yourself stuck in front of your TV or computer for the rest of the night if you eat your evening meal with friends or family, you'll also go a long way in fostering healthy, loving relationships.

➤ **Don't use videos, television, or the computer as a baby-sitter for your kids.** Once in awhile all parents do it: Plop their kid down in front of *Beauty and the Beast* for the 49th time in order to take a little break themselves. But if you rely too much on an electronic baby-sitter, you'll be denying your child the kind of intellectual and emotional stimulation he or she needs, and yourself the joys of parenting.

The Least You Need to Know

➤ Electronic media can be habit-forming.

➤ Televisions, computers, and telephones provide easy, but often empty, distraction.

➤ There are lots of techniques available to help you break your electronic addiction and learn to use communication tools in life-enhancing, not life-detracting ways.

Part 6
Bad Habits and the Big Picture

What do you do if it's someone you love or someone you work with who has the bad habit: Your spouse's nail-biting is driving you crazy, your son's "little white lies" are starting to erode your trust, and your office mate's Internet cruising means nothing's getting done. How can you intervene in the most helpful and supportive way possible? We'll give you some tips.

Maybe, just maybe, you need more help in breaking your own bad habits than we can give you here. Breaking entrenched behaviors like the ones discussed in this book often require you to face difficult aspects of your present and past life. Knowing who to ask for that help, and how to accept it, is an essential part of the process of change.

Throughout the book, we hope we've helped you avoid developing new bad habits as you break the old ones. A habit you really want to be careful about is prostelytizing: trying to change the world—and this time we mean the WHOLE world. We'll help you channel this urge in the same positive way you've broken your own bad habit: with courage, good humor, and tenacity!

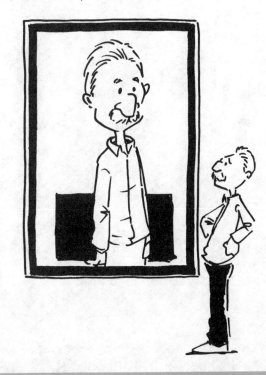

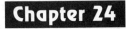

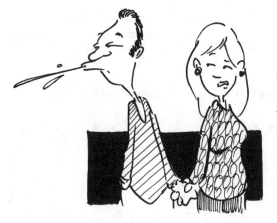

When Someone You Love Has a Bad Habit

The sound of another lie.

The sight of the constantly flickering television screen.

The smell of cigarette smoke.

The touch of a hand jittery from too much caffeine.

The taste of whiskey-stained lips.

Ah, love. It affects all of your senses, doesn't it? When you care about someone, whether it's a friend, a colleague, a partner, a sibling, or a parent, you notice everything about them, don't you? Even the annoying stuff. Maybe even especially the annoying stuff.

And there's the rub. Along with the way he smiles so sweetly comes the annoying way he has to chew every single bite of food exactly 20 times before swallowing. Not only does she have the best sense of humor in the world, she also grinds her teeth so hard at night, you think her head's going to explode (or yours!). Love someone, love their bad habit, or so it would seem.

No one's perfect, there's no doubt about it. Even you perform a behavior or two that annoys your nearest and dearest. We all do—that's part of life. When it comes to relationships, you've got to learn to accept the irritating with the charming, the unpleasant with the adorable.

The question becomes where you draw the line. How bothered are you by your loved one's bad habit? How much does it really disrupt your life or your loved one's life? Is the habit itself what's bothering you, or is the real problem something else about the relationship?

Should Love Be Blind?

In answering those questions, you've got to look once again at what a bad habit really is, and what role it's serving in your loved one's life—and in your own.

Let's face it: We all have behaviors that have the potential to annoy, and some of them we perform often enough to be called bad habits. In most cases, the people who love us endure our behavior, and now it's time for you to ask yourself if you can offer the same grace to the person in your life.

We have a friend who's best friends with her mother. She truly enjoys her mom's company, and especially loves going to the movies with her. But there's one thing that absolutely drives our friend insane: As soon as the last scene looks to be about over—but long before the credits begin to roll—her mother takes off her glasses, reaches for her handbag, puts on her lipstick, and gets ready to leave the theater. And every time she does it, our friend puts up with it and has an out-of-body experience.

Another friend named Evan is now divorced from a woman who had a gambling problem. At first, it was the attention it took away from their relationship that bothered him most. But then the electricity was shut off for non-payment, and the lies began to pile up, and pretty soon it was clear that his wife's behavior was out of control. Her bad habit was undermining not only her own goals, but his goals too and those they'd set together for their family.

Bad habits usually fall inbetween these two extremes. It's not something you can simply brush off with a grit of your teeth, but neither is it something terribly destructive like gambling, or full-blown alcohol or chemical dependency. It bothers you, and it bothers you for a reason. Before you can help your loved one break the bad habit, you've got to figure out just why it bothers you so much.

Remember, bad habits usually serve as a way to avoid or relieve stress and anxiety. If your partner sits in front of the TV every night and doesn't engage in a relationship with you or your children, it could be that he has more than a craving for reruns of serial killer movies and *Cheers*. Instead, he may be using television as a way to avoid his own feelings of anger, depression, or even a fear of intimacy. In some cases, there's also a level of passive-aggression involved: He might just be using the behavior, which he knows drives you crazy, as a way to express anger, or get back at you for things about the relationship he resents but won't discuss directly.

> ### A New Angle
>
> A 1995 study of adults found that 91 percent picked their noses on a regular basis. Now, if they'd only asked how many do so in public, we'd really have something to report!

It's what your partner's behavior is doing to your relationship that's the problem here, not the fact that the television is on all the time (and tell the truth, you kinda like *Melrose Place*, don't you?). Later in the chapter, we'll discuss how you can broach the subject of your loved one's bad habit and what's really at the root of it. In the meantime, it's important for you to find out how the habit makes you feel, how you respond to it, and what occurs because of the way you respond.

Denial Is More Than Just a River in Egypt: Identifying Your Coping Skills

How do you react when your loved one performs that annoying bit of behavior? Do you nag or sulk? Yell or give ultimatums? Ignore or deny it altogether? Or have you found supportive ways to work together to create a healthy atmosphere for change. Here's a quiz that'll help you identify the approach you take to your loved one's bad habit:

1. Your teenage son's room looks like a tornado hit it—for the umpteenth time. You respond by:

    (a) Persuading yourself it's not so bad.

    (b) Yell at him the moment he walks in the door.

    (c) Clean his room for him.

    (d) Make a deal that if he cleans his room every day for a week, he'll get to add another hour on to his curfew on the weekend.

2. Your husband comes home from work, and you can smell it on his clothes, though he swore he'd quit smoking two weeks before. You react by:

    (a) Convincing yourself the smell got there because a colleague smokes.

    (b) Snapping at him about how weak he is, then refusing to talk to him during dinner.

    (c) Never mentioning the incident, then sending his suit out to the cleaners.

    (d) Asking him what's going on in his life that's triggered his desire to smoke again, and what you both can do to relieve some stress.

3. You and your mother get in an argument over the phone, and she again tells you something you know isn't true. You respond by:

    (a) Telling yourself she simply made a mistake.

    (b) Calling her right back and accusing her of lying.

    (c) Telling yourself you provoked her behavior, again.

    (d) Calling her back and discussing the reasons why she felt it necessary to lie.

4. Your sister missed another family dinner because she lost track of time on the computer, which you know mostly involves "chatting" with strangers, but which she claims is work-related. You respond by:

    (a) Asking her how her work is going.

    (b) Refusing to invite her to Thanksgiving dinner.

    (c) Smoothing things over with the family by saying you forgot to invite her in the first place.

    (d) Offering to help her expand her social horizons by joining a gym with her or a lecture group.

5. Your colleague has terrible bad breath and you know it gets in the way of his professionalism. You respond by:

    (a) Telling yourself it's your imagination.

    (b) Giving him less interesting assignments and acting short with him in front of others.

    (c) Keeping him away from clients he might offend and conducting meetings with him over the telephone.

    (d) Alerting him, in private, to the problem.

How did you do? If you circled mostly...

A's, then you may be in denial. The way you're dealing with your loved one's behavior is simply pretending it doesn't exist. For awhile, denial appears to work, because it allows you both to avoid angry or embarrassing confrontations. In the end, though, denial keeps both of you stuck in the very same place: You feel resentful and helpless, and your loved one indulges in a behavior that perhaps undermines his or her health or future goals, and at the least threatens your relationship.

B's then you're reacting with anger and confrontation. And that's because you're pretty annoyed, aren't you? You've just about had it with your loved one's behavior, and you're not afraid to let him or her know that. Unfortunately, confronting your loved one with anger may only backfire. He or she may respond by rebelling—smoking, drinking, or lying even more just to assert independence. Or the feelings of belittlement and frustration could trigger the behavior by causing a rise in stress that the bad habit attempts to relieve.

C's, then you may be enabling, which means that instead of working toward changing unwanted behavior, your response allows it to continue. When your sister misses an important dinner because of a computer addiction and you smooth things over with the family, you're making it possible for her to continue her behavior without suffering any negative consequences. In fact, you're the one volunteering for the blame—how could you be so inconsiderate as to forget to invite your own sister to a family dinner? You become a guilty collaborator—*codependent*—in your sister's negative pattern of bad behavior.

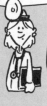

Strictly Speaking
Codependence is an emotional and psychological behavioral pattern by the spouses, parents, or friends of someone with an addiction or bad habit. This behavior "enables" the person to continue his or her negative habits.

D's, then you're being supportive, offering help in a gentle and encouraging way. As you may have guessed, the supportive approach is the only one that has any chance of succeeding. Next, we'll give you more tips on helping a loved one face a bad habit and then work to break it.

Stepping In, Gingerly

You don't know what to say or how to say it. You're afraid of the reaction you'll get. It's not the right time. There are lots of excuses, many of them valid ones, for not approaching your loved one about a bad habit. In the end, however, if the habit troubles you enough, you'll have to make the first move and air you concerns. Here are some tips to help get you started:

Cold Turkey
Leave the nagging behind! Nothing dampens a person's will to change faster than belittlement. Call a friend weak for having that second drink, and you might provoke a third or fourth. Flash "that look" when your significant other coughs "that cough" for the umpteenth time, and you may just find yourself eating alone at dinner.

Choose the right time, place, and mood. The time to discuss a loved one's tendency to release gas in public is *not* in front of company with anger in your voice. Instead, broach the subject when you're alone together, and calm.

Identify the bad habit. Believe it or not, some people don't realize they have a bad habit until someone points it out to them. They don't know enough about nutrition to choose the right diet or they think they're really not drinking so much. If your loved one doesn't believe that she or he performs the habit as often as you've witnessed, ask permission to keep a Daily Habit Log. Seeing it down on paper may help your loved one turn the corner. At the same time, keeping track could help you to appreciate when the bad habit is *your* problem and not your partner's. If your partner's tendency to pass gas in public bothers you, but not your partner or the people around you, and you see that clearly in the Daily Habit Log, you may be more willing to let it go the next time.

Express your concerns, gently. Without anger, without ultimatums, let your loved one know how the habit affects you and why you think it's important to break it. If you're worried primarily about her or his health, talk about it. But even if what's happening only affects the way you feel, you have a right to express that as well.

Ask how the habit affects your loved one. From your perspective, the fact that your friend is always late is an abomination. It embarrasses and upsets you, while it appears that your friend couldn't care less. When you talk about it together, however, you might find out that your friend's mortified, too, but just can't figure out how to be more punctual. Listen with your full attention to your friend's response to your concerns; it may help you know where to go from there.

Ask if your loved one's ready and willing to make a change. We know it's a cliché, but it's one that's got particular merit: People cannot change unless they really *want* to change. If your loved one doesn't truly believe that a bad habit is worth breaking, then all the nagging, cajoling, and negotiating in the world won't force a change. Asking is also a form of respect for your loved one's right to choose. Choice is a very important aspect of someone's life. If a bad habit has him or her out of control, giving them healthy choices—not ultimatums, remember!—can be the first step on the road to positive growth.

Find out how you can help—if you want to. If your friend decides that it's indeed time to make a change, let him or her know you're there for support and—if you decide you're willing—to provide practical help as well. Ask your friend to think about what you can do to help: Does he or she want on-going support or the opportunity to tackle it alone (for now)? Ask him or her to be as specific as possible about what's needed—and be as specific as you can about your limits. Setting compassionate goals, desires, and boundaries is a healthy start.

Decide what to do, for you. If your loved one isn't ready to change, you've got two options: You can decide to live with the bad habit, or you can decide to remove yourself from the relationship. The best way to make that decision is to perform a risk/benefit exercise as described in Chapter 6, "Step 2: Evaluate Risks and Benefits." If you get enough out of the relationship to continue despite the habit, then it's *you* who has to change so that you're not constantly under stress and annoyed. If you decide that your loved one's bad habit is simply too negative, then you should protect yourself and your sanity by getting some distance from the relationship for a short time. If you decide to leave the relationship altogether, make sure you get support from friends and counselors who can help you choose the best strategy for creating positive change in your own life.

Kids Do the Darndest Things

And the worst part of it is that they usually pick these darned things up from adults! Remember, most bad habits have roots in childhood; they developed as coping mechanisms in response to childhood anxieties and usually involve behaviors picked up through observation. Kids start throwing tantrums and being difficult all the time because they see their older brother or parent deal with stress that way. Or the bad habit can develop seemingly out of the blue, but in reaction to normal fears and anxieties of childhood.

What, you may ask, do children have to be anxious or fearful about? Think about it. The whole world is new and mysterious: the dark, strangers, feelings and emotions, you name it. Some bad habits kids develop in response to such stress may disappear as they grow out of a particular stage of development, or they may persist into adulthood.

In either case, your child's nail-biting, fibbing, or persistent sloppiness may well be driving you crazy. So how do you get him or her to stop? First, practice patience and offer love unconditionally. Know that there's at least a 50-50 chance that he or she will grow out of it before long. And finally, use these tips to get your point across:

➤ **Identify the behavior and discuss solutions.** Calmly point out what you don't like about the behavior and why. Say something like, "People don't take things that don't belong to them."

➤ **Involve your child in the process of breaking the bad habit.** If your child habitually twirls his hair or jiggles her knee, ask what other, less obvious behavior could be substituted. Make them think about it and encourage creative responses. Although deep breathing exercises may not seem to be appropriate for children, they truly can help break stress-related bad habits. Suggest that your child take slow deep breaths whenever he or she feels nervous, bored, or stressed. Make sure, though, that your child avoids holding his or her breath—that's not relaxing at all.

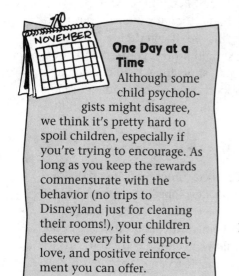

One Day at a Time

Although some child psychologists might disagree, we think it's pretty hard to spoil children, especially if you're trying to encourage. As long as you keep the rewards commensurate with the behavior (no trips to Disneyland just for cleaning their rooms!), your children deserve every bit of support, love, and positive reinforcement you can offer.

➤ **Reward and praise your child often**—and not only for efforts made toward breaking a bad habit. Congratulate your kid with a hug and a kiss for completing homework, for making you laugh with a joke, for just being a great kid. In addition, think of some specific rewards related to the habit: If he or she manages to stop sucking a thumb for a whole week, for example, allow an extra hour of television on a weekend night, or go together to the aquarium for a special afternoon. Don't worry, we know you'll think of plenty of loving alternatives that'll help your child grow up as healthy and strong as possible.

➤ **Keep lines of communication open.** What's important is constant communication and an atmosphere of trust. Kids can beat up on themselves enough, as well as run amok, without positive encouragement from their parents coupled with limits on their behavior that's clearly and firmly enforced.

Moving Forward Together

You wouldn't be reading this chapter if you didn't think, in your heart, that you could help someone you love along the road of change. As long as you don't end up giving more of yourself—emotionally, financially, or physically—than you can afford, we think you're right.

Two heads *are* better than one, and that goes double for two hearts. If you work together toward the same goal, the road will be a lot less lonely for the both of you. Once you're in agreement that change is what's needed, hand this book over to the person you love so much and then let nature take its healthy course!

The Least You Need to Know

➤ Bad habits can affect the ones you love and know best.

➤ There are positive and negative ways to intervene when trying to help someone you love break a bad habit.

➤ Offering positive reinforcement is the best way to help a child break a bad habit.

➤ You can move forward together toward a habit-free future.

Chapter 25

Knowing When You Need More Help

In This Chapter

➤ When it's more than just a bad habit

➤ Where to go for help

➤ Accepting support and moving forward

"Pull up your bootstraps." "Knuckle down." "Just think positive." "Be an adult." "It's just a matter of willpower."

How many times have people made statements like that to you during your struggle to break your bad habit? How many times have you said them to yourself? As Americans, most of us have been brought up to believe we should be able to handle our problems all by ourselves, on our own, "in the family."

We all may enjoy watching *Oprah* or *Ricki Lake,* but those public displays ironically make it harder for some of us to talk about our problems—we don't want to be vulnerable in front of a viewing audience! Asking for help, and then accepting it, continues to go against our national grain—now more than ever.

The Fine Line Revisited

But sometimes outside help is absolutely necessary. And how do you know if you've reached that point? Unfortunately, there's no easy formula we can offer you to answer that question—except to restate the obvious: If you think you need help with your bad habit, you probably do.

Before we go any further, though, give yourself another really big pat on the back. Just having the courage to admit that your problem might be too big for you to handle on your own is a great achievement. And you're continuing to look for answers. Congratulations!

In Chapter 10, "Identifying Your Cravings," we offered you a quiz designed to evaluate whether or not your bad habit had become an addiction. Your answers to those questions should help you judge your need for outside intervention. We've modified the questions just a little to put them into the proper context:

1. Do you indulge in your habit more than you intend to on a regular basis?
   *Yes*____ *No*____

2. Have you tried to break your bad habit before, but continue to be overwhelmed by persistent urges to indulge? *Yes*____ *No*____

3. Do you give up other things in order to indulge your habit? *Yes*____ *No*____

4. Do you continue on a course of negative behavior, even though you know it's doing harm to you and/or your relationships? *Yes*____ *No*____

5. Have you ever felt symptoms of withdrawal or overwhelming feelings of anxiety, sadness, or depression when you've tried to stop performing your habit?
   *Yes*____ *No*____

6. Do you need more and more of the substance or behavior to achieve the same level of pleasure or satisfaction? *Yes*____ *No*____

If you answered "yes" to any of these questions, then you just might need some guidance and support. You're clearly fighting a powerful enemy, one that's more than just annoying to you and the people around you. This enemy could be undermining your personal relationships, career, self-esteem, and very possibly your health. It also triggers cravings and urges you're unable to control, which means it's become a problem you probably can't handle on your own.

This Is More Than a Bad Habit, This Is a Problem

When you tried to quit, were you flooded with feelings that troubled you enough to fall into your old patterns? Remember, bad habits develop out of a deep-seated need to avoid uncomfortable feelings, thoughts, and memories. Your bad habit seemed like the best response to an overwhelming situation, until you realized that it was actually undermining your goals and sense of self-esteem. But until you address what's behind your habit, you may well remain caught in its grip longer than you need to be.

Or maybe you've even succeeded at breaking your bad habit, but at too high a cost. Are you now so tense and anxious you've got trouble getting through your day? Do you feel worse now than you did when you still had your habit? That may be because the feelings your bad habit allowed you to avoid are still there, working at you in full force, and now you've got no way to relieve the anxiety they cause you. Simply put, if you take away the habit, you're left with those uncomfortable feelings.

For many of us, that's when the real work begins—and where therapy can be of great value. Often, an objective person—a person outside our intimate circle of family, friends, and coworkers—can help us explore how we got to this point in our lives, and how we can move forward.

> **Cold Turkey**
> Denial ain't just a river in Egypt! If you suspect your bad habit is undermining your health or disrupting your relationships, don't wait until you've "hit bottom" to break the negative cycle. Reach out to your doctor, religious counselor, or trusted friend and admit you need help as soon as you can.

To Be in Therapy or Not to Be in Therapy: When a Therapist Can Help

Perspective and guidance: That's what a therapist is trained to provide his or her clients. By asking questions and listening with care to the answers, a therapist can see the connections—between the past and the present, between thoughts and deeds, and between emotions and reactions—that you're simply too close to the situation to recognize yourself. You've been living with and within your own behavior for so long, and your defenses are so high, that you need someone with training and vision to explore this new terrain with you.

As you've discovered by now (we hope!), bad habits often exist within a vicious cycle. You smoke as a way to soothe stress, relieve boredom, or to keep at bay feelings of insecurity or loneliness. But then there're the after-effects: You're nagged by your friends, you feel weak and afraid, and so you take another smoke to stuff those feelings down.

One of Gary's clients, an obese woman named Cathy, went into counseling not because of her weight, but because her husband no longer responded to her and had begun to get involved in outside activities he didn't share with her. With Gary, Cathy talked about what it meant to feel left behind, and in doing so, realized that she'd always expected her husband to reject her just the way others had rejected her in the past. That fear caused her to overeat, as a way to comfort and calm herself. Eventually, Cathy saw the role her weight played in fulfilling this negative expectation by driving a wedge into her marriage. Without talking to Gary, Cathy may never have seen the connections between her behavior and the potential ultimate outcome.

269

In addition to providing perspective, a therapist can also serve as your partner and helpmate as you struggle to change. He or she can provide tips like the ones you've read in this book to help get you through the process, and then help you adapt them to suit your individual needs. As you work on breaking your bad habit, your therapist can be your coach, preventing you from beating yourself up, encouraging you to continue, and helping devise new strategies for positive growth and change in your life.

Choosing the Right Kind of Therapy for You

Freudian analysis, interpersonal therapy, cognitive-behavioral therapy…there are any number of psychotherapeutic techniques, each with a different approach to uncovering underlying emotional problems and working toward a resolution. Fortunately, there's no need for you to choose among them, because most mental health professionals today are trained in a variety of techniques and draw upon a variety of approaches in treating each patient.

Finding a Therapist and Dealing with Insurance

How should you decide what type of therapist to choose? And what individual among that group might be right for you? These days, it's probably wise to start by checking with your medical or health insurance plan to see if it covers mental health services and, if so, how you may obtain these benefits. Many policies have arbitrary limits and may only cover 50 percent of the costs of a fixed number of visits per year. If you're one of the increasing numbers of Americans who is a member of a health maintenance organization, for example, you may be limited in your freedom to choose who can treat you and how long your therapy can last.

Strictly Speaking
Cognitive-behavioral therapy is a psychological approach that recognizes the complex interrelation of thoughts and behavior. It aims to identify and change distortions and thinking, as well as teaching you to substitute healthier ways of behaving.

If you have funds available, you may want to seek care outside your HMO or managed care plan. Many therapists offer a sliding fee scale based on your ability to pay. Mental health clinics and universities also extend low-cost therapy options.

After you know from what pool of therapists you can draw, ask your primary care physician to recommend who among them might be right for you. Ask for a couple of suggestions, as well as a copy of your medical records, so that the therapist can examine them at your first appointment. If you feel comfortable, ask friends and family for suggestions as well. Your local medical or psychiatric society are also good sources (see Appendix A, "More Bad Habit Busters").

You can choose from among the following mental health professionals:

➤ **Psychiatrists** are medical doctors who specialize in the diagnosis and treatment of mental or psychiatric disorders. In addition to providing therapy, psychiatrists can also prescribe medication. In some cases, especially in HMOs or other managed care situations, however, psychiatrists don't provide ongoing therapy.

➤ **Psychologists** have completed a graduate program in human psychology that includes clinical training and internships in counseling, psychotherapy, and psychological testing. Qualified psychologists may have a Master of Science degree (M.S.) or Ph.D. Psychologists don't have medical degrees, nor can they prescribe medication.

➤ **Social workers** (C.S.Ws, [certified social workers], or L.C.S.Ws [licensed certified social workers]) have completed a two-year graduate program with specialized training in helping people with emotional problems.

In addition to having proper credentials, the therapist should also have experience in treating men and women with problems similar to your own. If you've got a bad habit related to food, for example, you might want to find someone who's treated men and women with weight problems or eating disorders in the past.

How Therapy Can Help You Break Your Bad Habit

When it comes to helping you break your bad habit, there are a few different approaches a therapist may choose depending on the your particular needs. In some cases, he or she might use a very "here-and-now" technique, focusing on current relationships, career challenges, and family dynamics. Others will concentrate more on your past, looking for connections between what happened then and your present situation. A good therapist will be flexible, adopting multiple viewpoints depending on where you are in the process and what new challenges come up in your life.

One of the most helpful methods for dealing with bad habits is behavioral therapy. The theory behind behavioral therapy is that distressing, negative behaviors are learned responses that you can modify or unlearn, and by doing so, also change the way you think and feel. One basic technique of behavioral therapy is behavior modification, which aims to reduce or eliminate a bad habit by using reinforcement: that is, rewarding a desired behavior or punishing unwanted ones. The idea of putting gold stars on your calendar for every day you successfully cope with your habit is an example of a behavior modification technique.

Some therapists will be quite involved in your day-to-day progress, making specific suggestions about what you can do about breaking your habit and other aspects of your life you're eager to change. Others will be less involved, gently guiding and supporting you, but allowing you to take the lead.

271

No one technique is better than another—except in how you react to it. What's important is that you're comfortable with the approaches your therapist takes, as well as the rapport that develops between you. Does he or she seem to understand you? Is he or she empathetic? Are you comfortable sitting alone in a room with the therapist? Only you can answer these essential questions, and if you can't answer them affirmatively, then keep looking until you find a therapist you feel comfortable with.

One Day at a Time

Keep an open mind about your therapist's suggestions—as long as they're within professional boundaries. For example, talk about attending group therapy sessions if he or she suggests it, even if you're a little uncomfortable in a group. You might just learn something about yourself by confronting your fears and, eventually, sharing your experiences with others by joining a group.

In the end, no matter who you choose or what approach you take, you and your therapist should work toward these three basic goals:

➤ **Feeling better.** Chances are, you're feeling frustrated, sad, even weak. One of your first goals, then, should be to alleviate these feelings until you feel strong and confident enough to move forward. If you suffer from depression or an anxiety disorder—frequent cohorts with entrenched bad habits—the therapist may suggest a short term of medication to help you break the cycle.

➤ **Identifying sources of stress or unhappiness and tracking your progress.** Oh yes, a good therapist may very well ask you to do what we've suggested so many times: Keep a Daily Habit Log in order to identify what's triggering the feelings of stress that your bad habit helps to stave off. He or she can then help you translate that information into something you can use.

➤ **Making an accurate appraisal of your current situation.** Your inability to get a handle on your bad habit may make your life seem out of control and unmanageable. Maybe you think you've damaged some of your relationships beyond repair. A therapist will help you to more objectively assess what in your life needs fixing, and what's more on track than you think.

➤ **Identifying and changing self-defeating thought patterns and behaviors.** If you're like most people with ingrained bad habits, you've made a kind of internal audiotape of self-criticism and pessimistic thoughts. One of the most important goals of therapy is to erase this tape and make a new one filled with more positive, self-affirming thoughts.

➤ **Rebuilding self-esteem.** Therapy can help you identify your strengths and minimize your weaknesses, while helping you to see how worthwhile your struggle to change really is.

Some therapists like to treat their patients individually, and you may be asked to come once or twice a week for a 45- or 50-minute session. Others like to form groups of patients with similar, or even very different, problems. Both of these approaches have their merits and can be equally effective, but again it depends on what you expect from, and how comfortable you feel with your therapist.

Twelve Steps and Beyond

Individual and group therapy aren't the only—nor always the best—choices. Maybe you can't find a qualified therapist with whom you feel comfortable, or maybe your insurance program doesn't cover therapy and you can't afford private care.

Or maybe one-on-one interaction just isn't for you, and you thrive instead inside a solid support group made up of people coping with similar challenges—even the very same bad habit. Meeting with them on a regular basis can help you gain new perspectives on your habit, offer you suggestions and tips to help you break it, and shed light on a variety of other aspects related to the process of change.

The most well-known support groups are those based on the 12-step approach, such as Alcoholics Anonymous and the groups modeled after it, including Overeaters Anonymous, Gamblers Anonymous, and Narcotics Anonymous, among others. The basic premise of 12-step programs is that addiction is a disease and that total abstinence from the negative behavior or substance is essential. In fact, the first step is to admit that you're powerless over your addiction. Other steps and traditions emphasize self-honesty, humility, self-care, and group support.

In addition to 12-step programs, many other types of self-help groups now exist for people dealing with similar challenges to share their thoughts and experiences with one another. Often these groups don't have a professional leader or formal structure, and their primary goal is to provide support and encouragement, help you overcome a sense of isolation, and disseminate information. We list some of those resources in Appendix A.

A New Angle

An estimated 12 to 14 million Americans belong to support groups. In addition to Alcoholics Anonymous, Narcotics Anonymous, and others related to breaking addictions, support groups are also available for people with serious or chronic illnesses like cancer and arthritis, or for people who share a common challenge, like mourning the death of a loved one. Support groups offer empathy, compassion, and a sense of community and purpose.

Finding the Courage Within You

Admitting that you may not have the personal resources to kick your habit without help is a sign of strength, not weakness. It means you're willing to do whatever it takes to break a habit that's undermining your life, disrupting your relationships, and wreaking havoc on your self-esteem. By taking this next step, you're telling yourself you're worth the effort it takes to move forward.

That's not to say you won't have to work, and work hard. A therapist and a support group can help immensely by providing you perspective and guidance, but it'll be up to you to put the knowledge you derive from them together with the power that lies within you to move you forward to a brighter, habit-free future.

The Least You Need to Know

➤ You might need some help in breaking your bad habit.

➤ There's often a fine line between a bad habit and a serious addiction.

➤ One-on-one therapy can provide a new perspective on past challenges and future goals.

➤ You have millions of fellow travelers along the road of change. Sharing your experiences with them, and hearing their stories and suggestions, in support groups can help you on your journey.

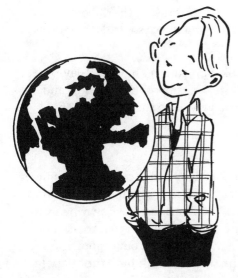

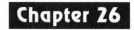

Chapter 26

Changing the World

In This Chapter

➤ Congratulations!

➤ Setting a proper example for others

➤ How to look beyond yourself

You've done the unthinkable, unimaginable, unfathomable. You've looked your bad habit straight in the eye and said, "This town isn't big enough for both of us." Ready or not, you've decided to part ways with your old bad habit friend and start down a new road. We applaud your efforts to "take life by the lapels," as poet Maya Angelou once wrote, and risk the process of change. *Carpe diem!* Seize the day! Enjoy the present.

Congratulations!

Making the decision to embark on a journey of change is courageous, exciting—and tough. Sometimes the bad habit you know seems more familiar, and therefore safer, than an unknown future filled with *unfamiliar* signposts. But as former U.S. President John F. Kennedy said, "Change is the law of life." And to go a step further, Muhammad Ali said, "The person who views the world at 50 the same as at 20 has wasted 30 years of life." Life is about discovery, and you're about to learn all kinds of new things about yourself by facing and overcoming your bad habit. You may even be surprised at the direction your efforts take you. Maybe you'll end up changing and growing in ways you'd never expect and you can't even begin to predict right now.

Remember what we said at the beginning of this book, Rome *wasn't* built in a day. You won't break your bad habit overnight. But with persistence, support from friends and family, and your trusty Daily Habit Log, you're off to a very good start!

Bad Habit Time Bombs

As you make progress in breaking your bad habit, you'll begin to notice a lot of people in the world around you who are stuck in bad habit ruts. You'll notice that clump of smokers standing outside the office building at lunchtime. You'll raise an eyebrow when your significant other would rather spend two hours participating in online chat rooms and scarfing down take-out rather than talk to you over a quiet dinner. You'll spot the co-worker who looks *fabulous* in haute couture—but who surely doesn't have the salary to match.

Bad habit time bombs are everywhere and your extra-sensitive habit radar system will detect them with greater frequency than ever before. "Wow, how do these people get away with it?" you'll wonder. Well, they're doing it the same way you used to—one day at a time, clutching their bad habits like talismans against a harsh, stress-filled world.

One Day at a Time

When you're mindful, you're fully experiencing all of your senses, feelings, and thoughts as you perform a task or activity. Try mindful eating. Feel the weight of the food on your fork, look at the food, taste it, concentrate on each bite. Feel your throat muscles contract as you swallow. Notice the fullness as your stomach accepts the food. Think about everything that has to do with eating, as you're doing it. Mindfulness makes every moment count.

It may be easier or harder for you to deal with the bad habit time bombs you encounter on a daily basis as you're working to break your *own* nasty behaviors. Some days you might feel smug and superior. Other days you might have the urge to run full tilt in the other direction—that baby's going to blow and you don't want to be anywhere in the vicinity! And yet there'll probably be days when you'll feel temptation beckoning and the tick of that bad habit time bomb will sound more like the reassuring rhythm of a heartbeat. After all, everyone's got at least *one* bad habit, right?

Here's the point. You'll have highs and you'll have lows. But if you're disciplined enough to stick to the program, they'll even out and you'll learn that just because your mind presents you with a strong emotion, craving, or bad habit urge in any given moment, it doesn't mean you have to act on it. Let the thoughts pass in and out of your mind and consider them as a detached observer might. Separate your thoughts from who you are and then decide which ones you like—and which ones you don't.

Instead of thinking about a million things all at once, focus on what you're actually doing, feeling, and experiencing in the moment. If, for example, you need an afternoon boost and you head for the coffee pot without even thinking, well, start thinking. Do you *really* want that coffee? Or are you bored, or do you just need a five-minute break from the task at hand? What's really happening? This is called *mindfulness*, and it's taught in many Eastern philosophies and used in stress-management clinics like the one at the University of Massachusetts Medical Center run by best-selling author Jon Kabat-Zinn.

Creating Change: One Habit at a Time

If you're like most people, you've actually got *more* than one bad habit. As you achieve some success at breaking the one, others may rear their ugly heads and demand attention. Gee, you might think to yourself, "That glass of wine really isn't so much fun without that cigarette." Gradually, you'll find yourself examining other areas of your life from a fresh perspective, and perhaps continue the process of change. Change is creation, and that's what you're doing: Creating a new you every day. You'll find yourself exploring new interests, meeting new people, and accepting new challenges. And all without your bad habits to hold you back!

Or, maybe the changes you're making will begin to affect your relationships with others; if you're making progress at controlling your temper, you might be surprised to find that your assistant at work is suddenly showing up on time, even early, instead of half an hour late every day. Or that instead of high-fat processed foods in front of the TV, your significant other is making nutritious gourmet meals to enjoy with you for cozy dinners at home. Breaking your bad habit may help you strengthen your relationships with others and bring you closer than ever to the people you care about the most.

Who knows, your positive example may help others decide to try breaking their bad habits, too! That person who was teasing you about the baggie full of "rabbit food" and your "woo-woo" yoga class is now envious of your healthy physique, your boundless energy, and your steady, unflappable calm in moments of stress. It could happen.

The Urge to Proselytize

But hold your horses! Don't go overboard and start pushing other people too much. Being nagged to break a bad habit, or constantly reminded of how well you're doing with breaking *your* bad habit, may make a loved one feel more like they're walking the plank or being pushed off a cliff than like they're receiving your help and respect.

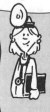

Strictly Speaking
Arrogance is the off-putting display of exaggerated self-importance or self-worth, and shows more pretension than substance.

Cold Turkey
Avoid **proselytizing**—attempting to recruit or convert others to an idea, belief, or activity that you've been recruited for or converted to. As you've discovered, the process of change must begin from within. Until your loved one is ready, proselytizing may only seem like nagging.

Arrogance is not the most attractive quality a person can have. And it isn't one you can afford when it comes to breaking bad habits. We're all in the same boat: We're all human, and we're all doing our best to be happy in life. We're all created equal—no matter how many or what kind of bad habits we have! So look with compassion on your bad habit fellows: You've been there. And you could be there again. That's another way of saying be nice to people at the bottom or the middle of the ladder because you might just meet them again on your way back down! Those people you're discounting today may be the very ones you'll depend on to help you through a tough spot or relapse tomorrow.

Instead of nagging or even "encouraging," try a more subtle approach. Research reveals that the most powerful messages are nonverbal ones. We first understand the visual (what we see), then move on to the auditory (our tone of voice), and only last do our brains register the meaning of spoken words. So it's really true that actions speak louder than words. And that people learn best by example. Instead of *proselytizing*, go about the business of breaking your bad habit, growing stronger every day, living without the burden that once held you back. People will see. And they'll get the picture all on their own.

Good Community Habits

We're going to quote JFK again. Can you guess which words we'll invoke? You got it: "Ask not what your country can do for you. But what you can do for your country." Powerful words when they were spoken back in the early 1960s, so powerful they stirred our nation to action. And they're no less powerful words today. The sentiment is one that's simple, but profound: Look beyond yourself. Look to your family and friends, your neighborhood, your town, your state, your country, your world.

When we feel good about ourselves and our inner strength, we have the energy and compassion to look outward. We have the vision to realize that we're all part of a community, one that in the twenty-first century will reach clear around the globe. Like Jimmy Stewart in *It's a Wonderful Life,* we realize that the richest person in town is the one who's given the most of him or herself.

A New Angle

Volunteering is making a comeback: According to recent statistics, about 95 million Americans volunteer every year. The average amount of time donated is about 4.5 hours per week—or a total of about 20 billion hours a year!

In breaking your bad habit, you're learned a lot about what it means to be human. You've got a lot to share with others:

➤ You know how fragile, and how strong, human beings can be.

➤ You've learned that by examining your life, you can make positive changes by understanding why you do the things you do.

➤ You're beginning to lend more than just a sympathetic ear to those around you; you're doing your best to empathize with others, acknowledging their viewpoints, feelings, and needs.

➤ You're no longer bored, stressed-out, and anxious all the time. You're challenged, hopeful, and ready for anything!

There's a wonderful Native American saying, "If the path has a heart, then keep walking." We hope you experience peace, health, and happiness on your life journey. And we wish you the best in breaking through any bad habit barriers you encounter along the way!

The Least You Need to Know

➤ Congratulations! You've made the decision to break your bad habit.

➤ Change is a healthy and inevitable part of life. You have to make positive changes to grow and evolve.

➤ As you change, you'll discover things you might not expect, about yourself and about the world around you.

➤ Don't nag others to change. Let your positive example speak for itself.

➤ The strength and confidence we get from breaking our bad habits help us to look beyond ourselves with empathy and compassion.

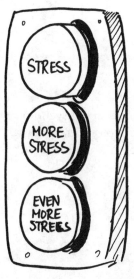

More Bad Habit Busters

The associations listed offer information, most of it free, about different aspects of breaking bad habits. In addition to their addresses and phone numbers, we also list (where applicable) their Internet addresses. Please be advised that many Web pages offer links to other sources of information, and that not all of these sources are reputable. Make sure you talk to your doctor or other appropriately licensed health care professionals about any issue, treatment, or theory that interests you before you assume that it has merit or is right for you.

General Mental Health Resources

As we've discussed, bad habits usually develop as a way to ward off anxiety, depression, or other uncomfortable feelings. In some cases, you may benefit from help provided by a mental health professional. The following organizations will provide you with further information and referrals:

> **American Psychiatric Association**
> 1400 K St., NW
> Washington, DC 20005
> (202) 682-6220
> Online contact: http://www.psych.org

The APA is a national organization of more than 40,000 mental health professionals. It provides information about mental health issues and referrals to the general public.

American Psychological Association
750 First St., NE
Washington, DC 20002
(202) 336-5500
Online contact: http://www.apa.org

The American Psychological Association is the world's largest organization of psychologists. It works toward the advancement of psychology as a science, a profession, and a means of promoting human welfare. It provides referrals and general information about mental health issues.

National Alliance for the Mentally Ill (NAMI)
2101 Wilson Blvd., Suite 302
Arlington, VA 22201
(800) 950-6294
Online contact: http://www.nami.org/

Founded in 1972 as a grassroots, self-help, support and advocacy organization, NAMI now includes more than 1,000 affiliated groups operating in all 50 states. NAMI provides free information on psychiatric illnesses, medicines, and financial concerns related to mental health care.

National Association of Social Workers
750 First St., NE, Suite 700
Washington, DC 20002
(202) 408-8600

The National Association of Social Workers is the largest organization of professional social workers. It is an organization that promotes, develops, and protects the practice of social work and social workers.

Anxiety Disorders Association of America
6000 Executive Blvd., Department A
Rockville, MD 20852
(301) 231-9350

A national network of consumers, health care professionals, and other concerned individuals, the ADAA offers a national membership directory, a self-help group directory, and a newsletter.

Alcohol-Related Problems

If you're having trouble controlling your drinking, there are several options available to you. First, visit your personal physician for advice and perspective. Psychological counseling may also be helpful. And if you still have concerns about your relationship to alcohol, or to someone who drinks, you can contact the following organizations:

Alcoholics Anonymous World Services, Inc.
Local branches nationwide—check your local phone directory
A.A. General Service Office
P.O. Box 459 Grand Central Station
New York, NY 10163
(212) 870-3400
Online contact: http://www.alcoholic-anonymous.org

Founded in 1935, Alcoholics Anonymous is a worldwide fellowship of men and women who have found a solution to their drinking problem. The only requirement for membership is a desire to stop drinking. The organization is supported by voluntary contributions of its members and groups, and neither seeks nor accepts outside funding. Members observe personal anonymity at the public level, thus emphasizing AA principles rather than personalities.

It is also important for you to seek help and advice from your family doctor or local hospital. You may require some medical help to break free of your addiction to alcohol.

Al-Anon Family Groups, Inc.
Local branches nationwide—check your local phone directory
1600 Corporate Landing Parkway
Virginia Beach, VA 23456
(804) 563-1600
(800) 344-2666
Online contact: http://www.al-anon.org/

If someone you love has a drinking problem, you'll probably benefit a great deal from the support and information provided by this offshoot of Alcoholics Anonymous designed just for people in your situation.

Help for Smokers

As tough as quitting smoking can be, there's lots of help out there. The following organizations offer support and information:

American Lung Association
1740 Broadway
New York, NY 10019
(212) 315-8700
Online contact: http://www.lungusa.org

The oldest voluntary health agency with 57 state associations and 60 affiliates throughout the United States, the American Lung Association provides help for smokers who wish to quit through the Freedom From Smoking self-help smoking cessation program—and you can do it directly on the Web at the above online address—as well as by contacting the ALA directly.

American Cancer Society
1599 Clifton Rd., NE
Atlanta, GA 30329
(404) 320-3333
Online contact: http://www.cancer.org

The American Cancer Society is a voluntary organization composed of 58 divisions and 3,100 local units. Through the "Great American Smokeout" in November, the Annual Cancer Crusade in April, and a variety of educational materials, ACS helps people learn about the health hazards of smoking and become successful ex-smokers.

Healthy Eating/Eating Disorders

It's hard to know the best way to eat and exercise. The following organizations offer information about these subjects, usually free:

The American Heart Association
7320 Greenville Ave.
Dallas, TX 75231
(214) 373-6300
Online contact: http://www.amhart.org

The President's Council on Physical Fitness and Sports
400 Sixteenth Ave., NW
Washington, DC 20036

Weight Watchers International
(800) 651-6000
Online contact: http://www.weight-watchers.com

This weight loss system emphasizes the importance of eating a balanced diet, one rich in fresh vegetables and fruits, as well as losing weight slowly and sensibly.

If you feel that your problems with eating go beyond what a little discipline and education can manage, contact:

American Anorexia/Bulimia Association, Inc.
293 Central Park West, Suite 1R
New York, NY 10024
(212) 501-8351

This organization offers information in the form of brochures and videotapes about eating disorders, as well as provides referrals to clinics, therapists, hospital programs, and support groups.

National Association of Anorexia Nervosa and Associated Disorders
Box 7
Highland Park, IL 60035
(847) 831-3438

This organization operates a phone line from 9 a.m. to 5 p.m. providing free information; telephone counseling; and nationwide referrals to therapists, support groups, and physicians who specialize in eating disorders.

Compulsive Behavior

Obsessive Compulsive Foundation
P.O. Box 79
Milford, CT 06460
(203) 878-5669
Online contact: http://www.pages.prodigy.com./alwillen/ofc.html

Founded in 1986, the OC Foundation is a worldwide nonprofit organization that provides referrals to both mental health centers and professionals, as well as coordinating support groups.

Financial Support

Debtors Anonymous General Service Board
P.O. Box 400
New York, NY 10063
Hot line: (212) 842-8220

Debtors Anonymous offers advice and support to people who chronically overspend and/or have a shopping compulsion.

Gamblers Anonymous
P.O. Box 1713
Los Angeles, CA 90017
(213) 386-8789
Online contact: http://www.gamblersanonymous.org

Gamblers Anonymous is a fellowship of men and women with a desire to stop gambling who share their experience, strength, and hope with one another in an effort to solve their common problem.

Internet Addiction

Believe it or not, the only organizations now devoted to the growing problem of online problems are located online! Here's one—and there'll be more before you know it—that might help you identify your problem as well as offer you support in breaking your bad habit:

Internet Junkies Anonymous (IJA)
Online contact: http://www.cyberramp.net/~bam/links/01.html

IJA is a fellowship of men, women, and children who share their experience, strength, and hope so that they may recover from excessive Internet use.

Personal Relationships

Learning what's appropriate in your romantic and sexual relationships may be helpful if you have trouble identifying or establishing boundaries. This organization provides information about practicing safe sex and other issues:

SIECUS (Sexuality Information and Education Council of the United States)
130 West 42nd St., Suite 350
New York, NY 10036
(212) 819-9776
Online contact: http://www.siecus.org

SIECUS is a 33-year-old nonprofit organization dedicated to affirming that sexuality is a natural, healthy part of life. It develops, collects, and disseminates information; promotes comprehensive education; and advocates the right of individuals to make responsible sexual choices.

Relaxation/Yoga

Integral Yoga Institute
227 West 13th St.
New York, NY 10011
(212) 929-0586
E-mail contact: IYI@aol.com

Offers Hatha yoga classes as well as courses in meditation, relaxation, breathing, balancing the chakras (spinal energies), yoga for specific health problems, and yoga for stress management. Also offers a yoga teacher training curriculum.

Yoga Research Center
P.O. Box 1386
Lower Lake, CA 95457
(707) 928-9898
E-mail contact: yogaresrch@aol.com

A great clearinghouse for information about all aspects of yoga.

Yoyoga
Online contact: http://www.yoyoga.com

This site offers an online newsletter and question and answer forum, as well as useful audiotapes and books on meditation, massage, and yoga.

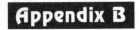

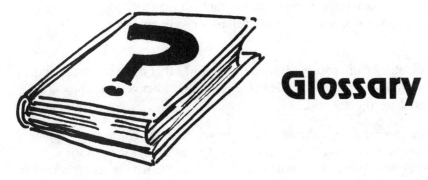

Glossary

In this section, we recap the definitions of some important words and terms about bad habits. We hope they help you in your quest for change and growth.

Absolute threshold   The minimum amount of stimulation it takes to create an urge or trigger a response. If your inability to resist a craving for a cigarette occurs after 10 minutes of stressful conversation with your boss, 10 minutes is your absolute threshold.

Addiction   Pattern of behavior based on a great physical and/or psychological need for a substance or behavior. Addiction is characterized by compulsion, loss of control, and continued repetition of a behavior no matter the consequences.

Alcoholics Anonymous   A worldwide organization that developed the first 12-step program for alcoholics based on group support.

Alcoholism   Chronic, progressive, potentially fatal disease characterized by physical dependence on alcohol, tolerance to its effects, and withdrawal symptoms when consumption is reduced or stopped.

Anhedonia   The inability to experience pleasure; a loss of interest in once-pleasurable activities.

Anxiety   Apprehension or uneasiness about an anticipated danger.

Attention Deficit Disorder (ADD)   A treatable neurobiological disorder characterized by symptoms of inattention, impulsivity, and oftentimes hyperactivity.

Avoidance   A psychological term used to describe the tendency many people use to stay away from situations that have made them uncomfortable in the past. You might well have developed your bad habit as a way to avoid feeling stress or anxiety in certain situations.

Caffeine   A drug, obtained from coffee, tea, and other drinks that has a stimulant action, particularly on the central nervous system. Caffeine is mildly addictive and is probably the most widely used drug in the world.

Cognitive-behavioral therapy   A psychological approach that recognizes the complex interrelation of thoughts and behavior. It aims to identify and change distortions and thinking, as well as teaching you to substitute healthier ways of behaving. This therapy is particularly useful in helping people break bad habits.

Cognitive dissonance   Psychological term that describes the difficulty that occurs when your attitudes don't match your behavior. It's uncomfortable—stressful—to accept both "I (an intelligent person) want to smoke" and "I know smoking is bad" as equally true. Instead, we alter one or another part of the equation: "Smoking isn't so bad" or "I'll quit tomorrow."

Compliance   The act of changing one's behavior to conform to outside pressure from family, friends, or community: Your spouse catches you in a lie and issues an ultimatum about lying. You comply—you stop lying—at least for a time, but don't really believe that lying is wrong.

Compulsion   A repetitive behavior that serves no rational purpose. Spending your entire paycheck on ceramic statues from a cable shopping network, despite the fact that you may not want to, is one example of compulsive behavior.

Craving   A deep yearning, longing, or desire for a particular substance. A craving can trigger habitual behavior, e.g., eating your third piece of chocolate cake.

Denial   A defense mechanism that allows a person to deny the existence of a behavior, thought, need, or desire in order to avoid the stress that would come from admitting it. You may deny that you crack your knuckles so that you can avoid having to stop driving your significant other crazy.

Displacement   A defense mechanism by which feelings are redirected from their true object to a more acceptable substitute. If you scream at the dog when your children are misbehaving, you're displacing your anger.

Freudian slip   Psychological term used to describe a behavior noticed by psychiatrist Sigmund Freud in which a person means to say or do one thing but ends up saying or doing something quite different.

Guru   A spiritual guide, taken from the Hindu meaning "dispeller of darkness." In today's world, *mentor* is the word we use to describe a teacher or other person who helps us grow personally or professionally.

Habit   A usual pattern of behavior that, over time, becomes ingrained and hard to change. Habits can be positive (brushing your teeth, saying "I love you" to your kids, exercising three times a week, etc.) or negative (smoking, biting your nails, overspending, gambling, etc.).

Impulsivity   Acting or speaking too quickly before considering the consequences of your behavior.

Internalization   The process by which a person incorporates a new attitude because it largely agrees with his or her system of values: You don't lie because you *know* in your soul that lying is wrong.

Internet   A network of information—social, financial, and general interest—that's transmitted electronically, over telephone cables through modems into computers. Internet addiction or overuse is a brand-new bad habit.

Limbic system   The part of the brain scientists believe controls or directs memory and emotion. It is made up of several different structures, connections, and neurotransmitters (brain chemicals) that work together. Many addictive behaviors are triggered, and then alleviated, by activity in the limbic system.

Maslow's hierarchy of motivation   Theory that ranks the human drives that must be fulfilled, usually in a specific order (although the hierarchy is dynamic), before humans can reach their full potential.

1. Physiological: Hunger, thirst, shelter, etc.

2. Safety: Feeling secure and protected from harm.

3. Social: Affection, acceptance, etc.

4. Esteem: Also called ego, esteem involves self-respect, achievement, recognition, status, etc.

5. Self-actualization: Achieving one's creative human potential.

Metabolism   The chemical and physical processes in living organisms involving the building up and breaking down of food.

Neurotransmitter   Chemical substance that carries impulses from one nerve cell to another. Dopamine, serotonin, norepinephrine, and adrenaline are a few examples.

Nicotine   A colorless, quick-acting poison in cigarette smoke. In small doses, nicotine has a stimulatory effect on the human nervous system. Nicotine is the most addictive substance in cigarettes.

Object permanence   Stage of development described by child psychologist Jean Piaget that occurs in infants between the ages of 18 to 24 months; the knowledge that an object continues to exist even when it's no longer perceived. That's how we know that the pizza we put in the refrigerator is still there.

Obsession   A recurrent, persistent, and senseless idea, image, or impulse; a thought not easily removed by thinking or talking about it. You can become obsessed with a person or sensation. If you act on the impulse, it becomes a compulsion.

Passive-aggressive behavior   The acting out of strong feelings in an indirect manner. Saying "No, no, don't bother. I'd rather sit in the dark," is a passive-aggressive way of getting someone to change the lightbulb for you.

Pleasure Principle   Psychological term coined by Sigmund Freud that refers to the natural impulse to avoid stress and pain at all cost.

Procrastination   Act of putting off doing something unpleasant or burdensome until a future time. Or the time after that.

Pyramid scheme   An illegal and fraudulent system of making money that requires an endless stream of recruits for success; also called a Ponzi scheme. Recruits must give money to recruiters and then enlist new recruits to give them money.

Reflex   Automatic reaction—physical or behavioral—in response to a specific action.

Relapse   The return of a behavior or habit after a person has quit. Relapse does not mean failure, but instead represents another opportunity to learn and move once again toward positive change.

Stimulant   A medication or chemical that increases brain activity. Caffeine and nicotine are stimulants, but for some, so are certain foods and certain behaviors that excite the central nervous system.

Stress   Any factor, physical or emotional, that provokes a response, positive or negative, in the body.

Tendency   An inclination to behave in a particular way; a leaning, bias, or propensity.

Transference   In psychology, a technical term for unconsciously bestowing upon another person the thoughts and feelings you normally associate with someone else in your life. For example, you unknowingly assign your feelings about your mother to your spouse or partner.

White lie   A term used to describe a lie about a trivial matter, often told to prevent or avoid conflict.

Index

When You're Smart Enough to Know That You Don't Know It All

For all the ups and downs you're sure to encounter in life, The Complete Idiot's Guides give you down-to-earth answers and practical solutions.

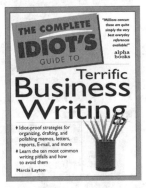
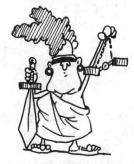
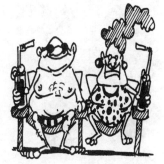
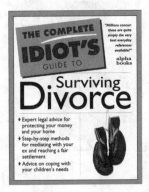

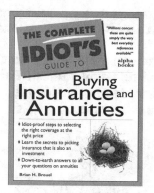
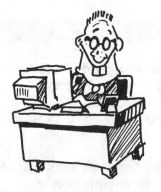
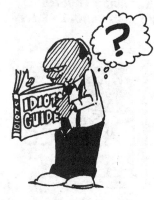
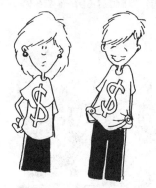
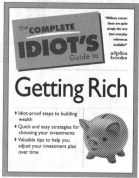

The Complete Idiot's Guide to Learning French on Your Own
ISBN: 0-02-861043-1 ▪ $16.95

The Complete Idiot's Guide to Dating
ISBN: 0-02-861052-0 ▪ $14.95

The Complete Idiot's Guide to Hiking and Camping
ISBN: 0-02-861100-4 ▪ $16.95

The Complete Idiot's Guide to Cooking Basics, 2E
ISBN: 0-02-861974-9 ▪ $16.95

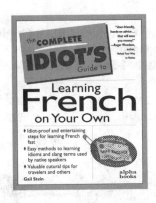

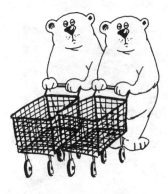

The Complete Idiot's Guide to Learning Spanish on Your Own
ISBN: 0-02-861040-7 ▪ $16.95

The Complete Idiot's Guide to Gambling Like a Pro
ISBN: 0-02-861102-0 ▪ $16.95

The Complete Idiot's Guide to Choosing, Training, and Raising a Dog
ISBN: 0-02-861098-9 ▪ $16.95

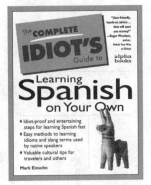

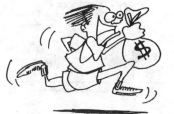

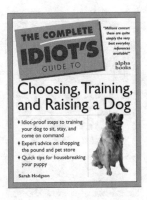

You can handle it!

The Complete Idiot's Guide to Trouble-Free Car Care
ISBN: 0-02-861041-5 ▪ $16.95

The Complete Idiot's Guide to the Perfect Wedding, 2E
ISBN: 0-02-861963-3 ▪ $17.99

The Complete Idiot's Guide to Trouble-Free Home Repair
ISBN: 0-02-861042-3 ▪ $16.95

The Complete Idiot's Guide to Getting into College
ISBN: 1-56761-508-2 ▪ $14.95

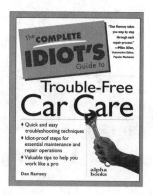

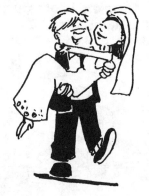

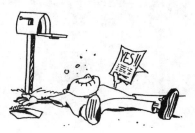

The Complete Idiot's Guide to Perfect Vacation
ISBN: 1-56761-531-7 ▪ $14.99

The Complete Idiot's Guide to First Aid Basics
ISBN: 0-02-861099-7 ▪ $16.95

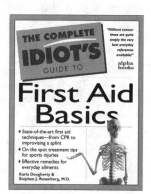

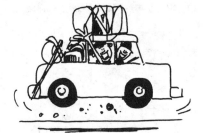

You can handle it!